Working With Fathers in Psychoanalytic Parent-Infant Psychotherapy

Working With Fathers in Psychoanalytic Parent-Infant Psychotherapy interfaces theoretical ideas about fatherhood and their incorporation into the clinical practice of psychoanalytic parent-infant psychotherapy. Often, when a family attends parent-infant psychotherapy, issues of the father are eclipsed by attention to the mother, who is usually the identified patient. Until now relatively neglected in the literature, this book attends to both the barriers to psychological work with the father, and to ways in which he can be engaged in a therapeutic process.

In this book, Tessa Baradon brings together some of the most eminent clinicians and academics in the field of parent-infant psychotherapy, in a layered collection of theoretical and clinical contributions. She and her co-discussants, Björn Salomonsson and Kai von Klitzing, conclude with an integration and critique of the themes presented, exploring the ideas of their fellow contributors and expanding on the central themes of the work.

Working With Fathers in Psychoanalytic Parent-Infant Psychotherapy will be of interest to mental health practitioners working with infants, who will learn that each individual and the family as a system can benefit from such an inclusive approach.

Tessa Baradon initiated the Parent Infant Project at the Anna Freud Centre and leads on the training in psychoanalytic parent infant psychotherapy at the Centre. She is Adjunct Professor at the University of Witwatersrand, School of Human and Community Development, and consults on parent-infant psychotherapy service development and training in different settings. She writes and lectures on applied psychoanalysis and parent-infant psychotherapy.

Working With Fathers in Psychoanalytic Parent-Infant Psychotherapy

Edited by Tessa Baradon

Discussants: Björn Salomonsson and Kai von Klitzing

Routledge
Taylor & Francis Group
LONDON AND NEW YORK

First published 2019
by Routledge
2 Park Square, Milton Park, Abingdon, Oxon OX14 4RN

and by Routledge
52 Vanderbilt Avenue, New York, NY 10017

Routledge is an imprint of the Taylor & Francis Group, an informa business

British Library Cataloguing in Publication Data
A catalogue record for this book is available from the British Library

Library of Congress Cataloging in Publication Data
Names: Baradon, Tessa, author.
Title: Working with fathers in psychoanalytic parent-infant psychotherapy / edited by Tessa Baradon.
Description: 1 Edition. | New York : Routledge, 2019. | Includes bibliographical references and index.
Identifiers: LCCN 2018043354 (print) | LCCN 2018058661 (ebook) | ISBN 9781315106830 (Master eBook) | ISBN 9781351605328 (pdf) | ISBN 9781351605311 (ePub) | ISBN 9781351605304 (Mobi/Kindle) | ISBN 9781138093454 (pbk.) | ISBN 9781138093423 (hardback) | ISBN 9781315106830 (ebk)
Subjects: LCSH: Parent-infant psychotherapy. | Father and child.
Classification: LCC RJ502.5 (ebook) | LCC RJ502.5 .B374 2019 (print) | DDC 618.92/8914–dc23
LC record available at https://lccn.loc.gov/2018043354

ISBN: 978-1-138-09342-3 (hbk)
ISBN: 978-1-138-09345-4 (pbk)
ISBN: 978-1-315-10683-0 (ebk)

Typeset in Times New Roman
by Swales & Willis Ltd

For my son,
And in memory of my father

Contents

Editor and contributor biographies ix
Preface xiii
TESSA BARADON
Acknowledgements xxi

1 A journey into fatherhood: the art of failing gracefully 1
DICKON BEVINGTON

2 The role of fathers in early child development 14
KAI VON KLITZING

3 'The door in the back of my head': a father's failure to mourn the deaths of his parents 28
ANGELA JOYCE

4 Waking daddy up: restoring a father's place in a borderline personality disorder couple 39
ALEJANDRA PEREZ

5 When working therapeutically with a baby's father is not possible 50
AMANDA JONES

6 Paternal orientations and the art of being a father 64
JOAN RAPHAEL-LEFF

7 Working with the triad 85
TESSA BARADON

8 The male therapist in parent-infant psychotherapy 94
ABEL FAGIN

9 The therapist and the father in parent-infant psychotherapy 106
YAEL SEGAL

10 Working with couples as parents and parents as couples 117
LOUISE EMANUEL

11 Can the difficulties of carrying out the paternal function for a toddler be identified from the earliest months of a baby's life? 124
MARIE-CHRISTINE LAZNIK

12 Freud on fathers: who cares? 139
BJÖRN SALOMONSSON

13 Three themes about fathers in parent-infant psychotherapy 154
BJÖRN SALOMONSSON, TESSA BARADON AND KAI VON KLITZING

14 And what about mothers? 169
TESSA BARADON

Bibliography 172
Index 185

Editor and contributor biographies

Tessa Baradon has been responsible for the development, implementation and evaluation of parent-infant psychotherapy services for high risk parents and infants at the Anna Freud National Centre for Children and Families, London, and has consulted on development of PIP programmes in the West and in developing countries, many of which are characterised by high community trauma. She is Head of Training of the specialist Psychoanalytic Parent-Infant Psychotherapy training at the Anna Freud National Centre for Children and Families, accredited by the British Psychoanalytic Council. Tessa writes and lectures on child analysis and parent-infant psychotherapy and has published extensively on these topics. In 2011 Tessa was appointed Visiting Professor at the School of Human and Community Development, University of the Witwatersrand (SA) and collaborates in research into cultural aspects of infant mental health.

Dickon Bevington is a father of three and consultant in Child and Adolescent Psychiatry. Prior to medical training in London, his first degree was in Anthropology, Comparative Religion and Philosophy at Cambridge. He works in the NHS in Cambridgeshire with young people who have complex needs including substance use, and as Medical Director of the Anna Freud National Centre for Children and Families.

Louise Emanuel was a Consultant Child and Adolescent Psychotherapist at the Tavistock Clinic in London and an Adult Psychotherapist in Private Practice. She was Chair of the Infant Mental Health Workshop at the Tavistock clinic for many years and also instigated the Brief Intervention Project to evaluate the effectiveness of brief psychotherapy with under-5s. She lectured widely in the UK and abroad and was the author of many peer reviewed papers. Louise was deeply involved in providing training and support to child mental health workers in the Townships of her native South Africa. She died in May 2017 after a short illness.

Abel Fagin is a Counselling Psychologist and works at the Parent-Infant Project at the Anna Freud National Centre for Children and Families where he delivers parent-infant psychotherapy and is part of the training committee for the Psychoanalytic Parent Infant Psychotherapy training. Abel is also employed at the Perinatal Parent Infant Mental Health Service at NELFT. He has a particular interest in working with adult mental health difficulties and Child Protective contexts.

Amanda Jones is a consultant perinatal psychotherapist and strategic and clinical lead of an NHS Perinatal Parent-Infant Mental Health Service. She trained as a systemic therapist and did her doctoral research at the Tavistock Centre/UEL. Her research studied how mothers' use of maladaptive defensive processes can derail their baby's development. In collaboration with the Anna Freud National Centre for Children and Families, Amanda was the therapist in the Channel 4 documentary series *Help Me Love My Baby.* With the NSPCC and Warwick Medical School she made five further documentaries called 'Breakdown or Breakthrough: pregnancy, birth and the first 18 months of life', available for free online, for all practitioners working with parents and babies in distress. Amanda speaks at national and international conferences on parent-baby disturbed relationships and psychodynamic parent-infant treatment.

Angela Joyce is a Training and Supervising Psychoanalyst with the British Psychoanalytical Society and a Child Psychoanalyst trained at the Anna Freud National Centre for Children and Families, London. There she was a member of the pioneering Parent-Infant Project for many years and also jointly led the child psychotherapy service. She works in private practice in London. She is currently Chair of the Winnicott Trust and a Trustee of the Squiggle Foundation and is an Honorary Senior Lecturer at University College London. She teaches widely and has written papers and contributed to books on early development and parent-infant psychotherapy, and Winnicottian studies. Her book edited with Lesley Caldwell, *Reading Winnicott*, was published in the New Library of Psychoanalysis Teaching Series in January 2011; she contributed the Introduction to volume 6 of *The Collected Works of D. W. Winnicott*, published by Oxford University Press in 2016; and she edited *Donald Winnicott and the History of the Present*, the papers from the London conference of the same name, published by Karnac in 2018.

Kai von Klitzing, MD, is Professor of Child and Adolescent Psychiatry at the University of Leipzig, Germany, and a psychoanalyst for adults, adolescents, and children. He is President of the World Association for Infant Mental Health, Editor of the *Journal Kinderanalyse/Child Analysis*, and Associate Editor of the *Infant Mental Health Journal.* His scientific interests include developmental psychopathology, early triadic relationships (mother-father-infant), children's narratives, psychotherapy (individual and family), childhood maltreatment and biological stress regulation. He has published books on attachment disorder, children of immigrant families, child psychotherapy.

Marie-Christine Laznik, PhD, psychoanalyst, member of the ALI (Association Lacanienne Internationale) and member of the board of the CIPPA (Coordination Internationale des Psychoanalystes, Psychothérapeutes et Professions afines s'occupant de personnes avec autisme). She has worked with adults in private practice and with children and babies for more than 40 years at Centre Alfred Binet, Paris. Laznik is author of the signs of the gride PREAUT: Signs of risk of autism at four and nine month, and trains child psychiatrists and psychotherapists in the « re-animation » of babies in danger of autism in France, Brazil and Morocco. She has written many books and articles on the subject.

Alejandra Perez is an adult psychoanalyst of the Institute of Psychoanalysis and a Parent-Infant Psychotherapist at the Anna Freud National Centre for Children and Families. She has done research on attachment, psychoanalysts' styles of working and systematic reviews for the NICE mental health guidelines. At present, she is researching mothers' experience of parent-infant observations. She is Programme Director of the MSc on Psychoanalytic Developmental Psychology at University College London and the Anna Freud National Centre for Children and Families, where she has taught psychoanalysis and led parent-infant observation seminars since 2008. She also has a psychoanalytic private practice.

Joan Raphael-Leff, PhD is a Psychoanalyst (Fellow of the British Psychoanalytical Society, Member IPA) and a Transcultural Social Psychologist. In clinical practice and academic research over the past 45 years she has focused on emotional issues of Reproduction (infertility, pregnancy, neonatal loss, early parenting), with over 150 single-author publications and 12 books in this field (translated into a dozen languages). Previously she was Professor of Psychoanalysis at Essex University, UK and led the University College London MSc in Psychoanalytic Developmental Psychology. In retirement she leads the Anna Freud National Centre for Children and Families Academic Faculty for Psychoanalytic Research and is consultant to perinatal and women's projects in many different countries, including South Africa where she was Professor Extraordinary at Stellenbosch University.

Björn Salomonsson is a training and child psychoanalyst of the Swedish Psychoanalytical Association, Stockholm, working in private practice and at the Mama Mia Child Health Centre. As Associate Professor at the Unit of Reproductive Health, Department of Women's and Children's Health, Karolinska Institutet, his research and publications focus on psychoanalytically inspired parent-infant therapies (theory, practice, and outcomes), child analysis, and the 'weaving thoughts' case presentation method. His books, *Psychoanalytic Therapy with Infants and Parents: Practice, Theory and Results* and *Psychodynamic Interventions in Pregnancy and Infancy: Clinical and Theoretical Perspectives*, were published in 2014 and 2018 by Routledge. A third book, written with Majlis Winberg Salomonsson, was published in 2016: *Dialogues with Children and Adolescents: A Psychoanalytic Guide* (Routledge).

Yael Segal is a clinical psychologist, training analyst at the Israel Psychoanalytic Society and a parent-infant psychotherapist. She is founder and director of the Ziama Arkin Infancy Institute at the Interdisciplinary Center in Israel. The Institute has clinical and research units and runs a two-year training programme in parent-infant psychotherapy. Yael also has a psychoanalytic private practice.

Preface

Tessa Baradon

Parent-infant psychotherapy is a treatment modality to address compromised interactions between parent and infant that may disturb the infant's developmental trajectory. In the early years of practice of PIP the mentors to our work at the Anna Freud Centre, such as Fraiberg, Cramer and Stern, helped us imagine our way into the exquisitely complex dances of the mother-infant relationship. With time, however, I noticed the absence of fathers in the consulting room even when they were, reportedly, active fathers in the home. This seemed puzzling, given the evidence that fathers are important to their children's development (see von Klitzing, Chapter 2 in this book) and that fathers in Western countries nowadays tend to be more involved in their babies' care. Furthermore, research suggests that these factors are related since nurturant fathering is constructed through increased caregiving activity (Abraham et al., 2014a). Discussions with colleagues yielded the same contradictory information: on the one hand, there is increasing awareness that 'Dads Matter' to their children's development, and that mental health difficulties in fathers impact their parenting and their children's and family's functioning (Ramchandani et al., 2011). Yet, on the other hand, fathers continue to be sidelined in the settings where services are provided to their infants.

A central contributor to the bias against fathers must surely be the dominant mother-centric theories of child development, including Attachment theory and research, and the historical socio-economic and cultural contexts in which these ideas were/are embedded. Additional explanations have been offered in the literature: men's own reluctance to seek psychotherapeutic help when in need (Addis & Mahalik, 2003), lack of recognition by professionals of psychological problems in fathers (Fitzgerald, Bocknek, Hossain, & Roggman, 2015), policy and systemic bias in programme development and delivery (Panter-Brick et al., 2014), and the attitudes of the individual delivering the service (Homberg & Olds, 2014). This book is the product of years of practice that actively seeks to overcome intrapsychic, interpersonal and organisational obstacles to accessing the fathers in families who seek help, and to include them in the therapy in their different roles.

The role of the father has undergone many socio-cultural and psychoanalytic iterations. Each, in my view, potentially adds a dimension to the complexity of father and fatherhood, rather than cancelling out previous conceptualisations. Classically, the cultural and psychoanalytic function of the father was that of bringing order through establishing boundaries and curbing the narcissistic omnipotence of the infant by setting limits to what can happen (barring incest). Whether the father's actions contribute to development depends on the way in which paternal authority is established and this, in turn, is affected by how the father has managed to integrate different aspects of himself. Frosch (1997) argues:

> to father a child requires something other than the traditional boundary-setting and prohibitive stance . . . but to reach out in a loving way requires a shift of masculine consciousness, involving not just some more gentleness but a whole gamut of *alterations in relations of dependency, intimacy, vulnerability and trust.*
>
> (p. 50, italics added)

The nurturant father, a more visible position socially today, can be viewed as someone who has better managed the conflict between maternal and paternal function in this role. Raphael-Leff (Chapter 6) describes this as the Reciprocator father, who can 'alternate between self and others to meet his own needs while nurturing another, but having to recognize needs different from his own'. When the father struggles to reach this position, we may see greater intrapsychic integration as an aim of therapy.

The perspective of the infant is also central to understanding the role of the father. Nurturance is seen to be doing things for the baby in line with father's personality and his imaginative understanding of his infant, which will differ to a lesser or greater extent from the way the baby's mother adapts and responds to her/him. In the context of the baby's *lived experience with both parents* when they are present to him, the 'genderedness' of 'father' is significant – not least in terms of the infant's (surmised) embodied and symbolic experience of maleness. The visceral experience of being handled and played with by a male parent and the quality of holding and separation offered by the father, will be woven into the particularity of each infant's experience of stimulation and sensuality. The *internal father of the child* develops from the interactions with the father when present in the child's life, but even an unknown or failing father exists for his child as an internal, psychic presence. The psychological consequences for the child whose father fails to fulfil his comprehensive roles is vividly captured in the clinical chapters in this book.

Intertwined with the exploration of fathering and impediments to it, is the question of triangulation. A comment on the terms 'triangulation' and 'triadification'. 'In family-systems literature "Triangulation" refers to a dysfunctional family processes wherein two persons in the family, frequently mother and father, manage their conflicts by pulling the third, often a child, into the process' (Bowen, 1978). Klitzing and colleagues (Klitzing, Simoni, & Bürgin, 1999) distinguish between triangulation – 'the interpsychic processes of experiencing a triad' (p. 3) and triadification, which are the interactive, interpersonal processes of forming a triad.

In this book the authors use to the terms interchangeably to refer to the capacity of each member of the family to enter a psychic triangular space. Britton describes this as tolerating 'the possibility of being a participant in a relationship and observed by a third person as well as being an observer of a relationship between two people' (Britton, 2004, p. 47). In my view, establishing triadic, as opposed to dyadic, relationships imply both the capacities for inclusivity and reciprocity between the three people.

It is the position of holding on to an internal notion of reciprocity while being an observer that seems particularly challenging with the birth of a baby. Becoming a family is a complex affair in which feelings of envy and exclusion are easily aroused. There are ghosts on the paternal as well as maternal side (Barrows, 2004) as well as cultural and systemic influences that need to be mutually accommodated. The therapy may address the couple relationship and/or co-parenting, with each carrying somewhat different positions for the baby. The couple relationship positions the baby as the third in relation to the sexual link of the parents, whereas co-parenting refers to presenting collaborative and respectful parenting to the child irrespective of the parents' coupledom. Von Klitzing discusses the importance placed in psychoanalytic literature of father claiming mother as his sexual partner: it relives the burden for the child of being her love object and lays the ground oedipal resolution. This issue is addressed also in Laznik's chapter and Salomonsson's discussion. Co-parenting is an issue that has been highlighted not only in the context of separated families (often to facilitate continued contact between father and child), but in the context of the intact nuclear family, since parental discord has such a negative impact on the children in the family (Holmes, Cowan, Cowan, & Hawkins, 2013). This was an integral part of the clinical work described by Perez and Jones.

Whereas in the past I have asked 'And what about fathers?' (Baradon, 2010), here we need to be curious about the mothers. The mother is critically important to the father's relationship with his baby. On the one hand, studies show that marital satisfaction and spousal support are more closely linked to fathering and father-child relationships than to mothering and mother-child relationships (Gordon & Feldman, 2008). On the other hand, mothers can be gatekeepers who regulate access both physically and psychologically. McDougall wrote

> a father who is physically present might nevertheless be lived as symbolically lost, absent or dead in the child's inner world depending once again on the father's own personality and *on the way the mother invests and speaks of him to the child.*
>
> (1993, p. 239, italics added)

Unconscious messages regarding the father are conveyed also in embodied ways. Slight pressure in mother's clasping of the baby as father approaches, or an open inclusive smile, are very different communications, even instructions, to the baby. Consciously available, and sometimes co-constructed, representations of father (e.g. as the incompetent parent) can influence patterns of behaviour; in clinical sessions, as in the home, a crying infant may automatically be transferred from father to mother for comfort. Querying this, the shared response was 'I'm not good with feelings' and 'He can't take the crying'.

Within the matrix of the therapeutic encounter, a fourth person enters the interactional system: the therapist. The authors who have contributed to the book share a psychoanalytic background, in which the co-constructed relationship between /therapist and patient is a central concern of the therapeutic process. The subjectivity of the PIP therapist in relation to the father and gender is also a subject of this book. As practicing professionals, our individual experiences indelibly influence the prism though which we approach our patients. In my family, generations of baby tucked to sleep in the crook of daddy's arm has led to a familial imprint, a visceral memory of the safety and physicality of daddiness, as well as to mnemonics of absence and of exclusion. Undoubtedly this contributed to my steadfast interest in babies and their fathers, fathers and their babies. In a professional setting, personal experiences and representations intertwine with transferences from the patients; assumptions – conscious or otherwise, frame and limit therapeutic hypotheses. These ideas are addressed, in one way or another, by all the contributors to this book.

The organisation of this book

The book is opened by Dickon Bevington's personal account of the slow recognition of the enormity of fatherhood and the turbulence of letting 'an other' and 'anotherness' into his life and coupledom and broader network of relationships. Starting with the personal 'completely-at-a-loss-ness' that parenting so often entails, Bevington considers the joy, brutality and terror at birth, the complex feelings of being 'quite exhausted, overwhelmed, and inadequate and worried about whether I could love the new baby'. Thus, Bevington personalises the theoretical and research knowledge that becoming a father is a central life event, triggering biochemical and psychological changes, and familial-cultural repositioning. Furthermore, his story illustrates some of the nuanced ways in which each father must assumes his fathering with each child.

In Chapter 2 Kai von Klitzing discusses research and psychoanalytic ideas on how the manifold changes that are associated with fatherhood are negotiated, and potential impact on infant outcomes. He discusses various levels through which a father may exert his influence: the real father, the father as part of the parent-infant triad and the internal father. Von Klitzing discusses the debate around gendered thirdness, and concludes that parenting is not gender neutral:

> the origins of life still have something to do with sexuality (in reality and or in the phantasies of the parents and the developing child), the parental behaviours are not independent from sexual instincts, and the relationships between the parental figures, and the ways in which these relationships are increasingly represented in the mental life of the child are not free from sexuality either (whether in primitive, more mature, or sublimated form)

Chapters 3 and 4 bring in the clinical work with fathers who are struggling to assume an active fathering of their infants when ghosts from their past meet with current traumatic circumstances.

Angela Joyce, in Chapter 3, notes that it was the mother who was referred as a source of concern but, it rapidly became clear to her that the father was also in difficulty. Joyce discusses the long reach of un-mourned loss of his parents in childhood, when he became a father himself. Explaining the occurrence of the après coup, Joyce describes how a traumatic birth of his baby evoked fears that he would lose his wife and baby and was marked by the phantasies associated with his parents' deaths. This father's long-standing defence to manage the unbearable, that of emotional shutdown, came into play also with his baby.

Alejandra Perez's case, in Chapter 4, discusses how '[t]he physical presence of the father may be neither sufficient nor necessary for triangulation to evolve' (Target & Fonagy, 2002, p. 57). Perez elucidates the ways in which characteristic BPD conflicts around difference and separateness were played out in the mother's demand for enmeshment with her baby and rejection of triangulation. These conflicts of his partner resonated with the father's own unresolved conflicts with his absent father in childhood. Both Joyce and Perez empathically describe how failing their babies was a guilt-evoking compromise solution to unbearable internal pressures.

In Chapter 5 Amanda Jones responds to situations where the father is not able to do the therapeutic work described in the previous chapters. Furthermore, his excessive use of splitting, denial and projection place the onus of dysfunction in the mother such that she may develop an emotional/psychiatric illness. Their baby is then at considerable risk. Jones advocates therapeutic work with mother and baby, even if opposed by the father, to help her understand her own psychic functioning – including its transgenerational origins, as well as that of her baby and partner. In her detailed case illustration Jones demonstrates speaking to mother as the baby (representing what she imagines the baby feels) in order help mother recognise the 'father-projected-into-the-baby's-mind' and free the baby from this experience.

Chapter 6 is positioned as a review and expansion on paternal mental states and functioning described in the chapters. Joan Raphael-Leff, in this chapter, addresses paternal orientations – 'patterns of being a father' – and contexts within which they develop. Multifactorial, external and internal cultures influence parenting patterns. In broad sweeps, but informed by both her research and clinical work, Raphael-Leff considers four paternal orientations which reflect the individual father's accommodation of his identity as progenitor, underlying anxieties and conflicts, and his 'act of acceptance' of fatherhood. Raphael-Leff then explores possible couple permutations inasmuch, she claims, paternal orientations have their maternal corollaries. Certain paternal orientations – such as the extremes of Renouncer and conflicted father, are often those encountered in the PIP consulting room.

In Chapter 7, I start a discussion about the challenges a therapist may face in working with the triad; this theme is continued in the chapters by Fagin and Segal. I describe the differences in positioning of each participant in PIP work with the triad. I suggest that the foursome of baby, mother, father and therapist constitutes a libidinal group, invested with the love and hate of a family group. But the therapist is an 'outsider within' and must contend with transferences and countertransference issues that attack on the group as an attachment unit. Another challenge to the therapist is that having the father, mother and baby together in the room potentially introduces sexuality very directly. It is concretely present in the existence of the baby and his/her bodily excretions, in the sensuality of care – such as breast feeding and can also be used defensively. In many ways, the impact on the therapist can be arousing, uncomfortable, threatening.

Abel Fagin, in Chapter 8, elaborates on some of these themes from the point of view of a male therapist. He contends that the gender of the therapist necessarily evokes a dynamic in the treatment and elaborates on some of the contradictory transferences and phantasies he has experienced as a male therapist. Fagin presents a case where he was experienced as nurturant by the couple and this enabled the father to reconsider his perception of emotionality and sensitivity as a weakness in men. In the second case introduced, Fagin was tasked with surviving the rage towards men of a single mother and holding a protective paternal presence. He describes some of the vicissitudes of eroticisation of the transference in both mother and daughter, and the challenges to remaining a reparative male figure.

Yael Segal, in Chapter 9, focuses mainly on transference-countertransference issues. She suggests clinical theory exists for mothering and the mother-infant relationship but is lacking with regard to fathers and the father-infant relationship. Consequently, clinicians are working in less chartered waters when it comes to understanding the manifestations of paternal subjectivity in the transference and their own biases in the countertransference. Segal illustrates her thesis through two cases in which paternal needs were obscured by the therapist's countertransference responses. In the first there was an enactment in which the father was excluded from the therapy by the therapist, and in the second the father's defensively sexualised transference was unbearable to the therapist. In both cases, these impasses were worked through by the therapist: in self-analysis (case one) and supervision (case two).

Louise Emanuel's contribution, Chapter 10, is the paper she gave at the WAIMH Conference in Prague in 2016. It was to be the basis of her chapter for this book but, unfortunately, she became ill before she could start this task. During her illness we discussed including her paper, despite its brevity, to represent her thinking and her work. Emanuel advocates the couple relationship as a key port of entry to addressing parenting difficulties and children's symptomatology. She links this with children's need for a combination of maternal and paternal functions, which can be embodied in parents of either gender, to flourish. Emanuel sees her role 'to help parents function as a "containing parental couple"' and illustrates her approach through clinical examples.

The last chapter in the theoretical/clinical contributions, Chapter 11, is by Marie-Christine Laznik, who presents a Lacanian view of the paternal function of nom de Pere. Laznik relates the story of a two-year-old whose father, in an attempt to distinguish himself from his own frightening father, tried to be his son's friend. Relinquishing all paternal potency and authority, he left his child psychically fatherless and consumed by annihilation anxiety: that he will be re-engulfed by his mother, without protection. A second case demonstrates the work to establish the law of the father and the psychological changes both parents needed to make for their baby to find 'a figure to embody the father in reality'. In explicating these dilemmas with the parents, Laznik herself models the third and how triangulation can function.

Laznik discusses the state of instinctual and relational disarray in the infant whose father absconds from his captaining his familial boat in the context of babies at high risk of autism. This calls to mind the family seen by Perez, where the baby started showing withdrawn, autistic-like states. The two analysts use different theoretical frames to understand the clinical material, but share the understanding about the pivotal role of the father in 'saving' the infant from engulfment by a phallic mother.

The final three discussion chapters represent our – the discussants – attempts at integration and critique of the themes presented.

In Chapter 12, Björn Salomonsson offers his thoughts on each of the chapters above. In structuring his discussion he has allowed it to flow associatively, yet clustered around certain themes, rather than systematically going through each chapter in sequence. This makes for a fluid experience in reading the discussion, as though wandering through the book in the company of another.

In Chapter 13, I explore the question 'and what about the mothers?' as gleaned from the discussions about the fathers. I suggest that whether a mother can support a role for the father is linked to her capacity for triangulation and the management of ambivalence within the triad.

Finally, Kai von Klitzing, Björn Salomonsson and I round off the book in Chapter 14, and explore three central themes that caught our imagination: is there a specific phenomenon of father's transferences? What kinds of intervention occur in therapies that are inclusive of fathers? What triadic capacities can be seen in PIP therapists?

Acknowledgements

This book follows my professional ‘developmental line’ from analytic work with individual child patient, to dyadic parent infant work, to working analytically with the triad. All along the way, patients and colleagues have been a cardinal to this.

Björn Salomonsson and Kai von Klitzing have given much thought and time to this this book and, consequently, it is all the richer. I have enjoyed our collaboration so very much on a personal as well as professional level.

Each chapter is an authentic contribution to the topic and reflects the integrity of the author’s work and thinking. Despite working individually on their chapters, as a collective of writers they generously considered not only their specific piece but the book as a whole, and worked around that.

The influences of the team of therapists and affiliated researchers in the Parent-Infant Project at the Anna Freud Centre infuse this manuscript.

Fathers and their partners and children – in my personal life, in the consulting room, the school-run in Hampstead, at the baby swings in playgrounds, and picnics on the local green have contributed to the sense that ordinary fathering matters, and thus figure in this book.

Chapter 1

A journey into fatherhood

The art of failing gracefully

Dickon Bevington

This chapter describes one father's now receding memories of coming into this role, something I'm blessed to have been able to navigate on three occasions, starting twenty one years ago. I can't begin to describe the gratitude I feel towards my children and their mother for giving me this opportunity, and apologise to them in advance for the misrepresentations that will inevitably follow in this account, let alone for the past decades. I have, however, tried to stick primarily to the brief of writing about *fatherhood*, and my own early encounters with it, so I have purposefully not written this chapter about them, but have focused instead on what happened inside and around me, from my perspective. This will, I hope, preserve their well-deserved dignity, but I can already hear at least one voice, perhaps a chorus, saying 'so it's all about you, Dad? Thanks'. I shall choose to hear that as containing one measure more of fond teasing than of straight out criticism. That's the thing about parenting (because I am assuming that mothers experience the same) it's a ride into at the very least uncertainty, but more likely towards certain failure. My aim is to make this just about fine, because that has been my experience.

I was relieved to be given a completely blank slate: '*impressions, not a thesis*'. I'm a child and adolescent psychiatrist in the NHS, where I work with adolescents with complex difficulties including problematic use of substances, and I also work as the Medical Director at the Anna Freud National Centre for Children and Families. Despite being in a trade which revels in building theories, gathering evidence, and all the rest of that wordy stuff, I have always rather tried (or at least intended) to avoid bringing my work home. Instead, without necessarily thinking it through too carefully, I suspect I sort of modelled myself on the kind of 'muddling through' that the poet Philip Larkin referred to as old-type and naturally fouled-up. I failed, of course, or succeeded, depending on which way you look at it.

One of the (very few) downsides of my professional role is finding oneself positioned as a parent who's actually expected to know about parenting and children. I know my work colleagues will understand the peculiar sting of hearing frank familial feedback on the gulf between that expectation and this reality; there is a world of difference between professional competence and the personal 'completely-at-a-loss-ness' that parenting so often entails. This perhaps begins to explain the 'failing gracefully' phrase in my title, but also reveals another happy failure of sorts, in that it's a phrase that arose and which I often use at work. I use it with parents, to describe (even prescribe) their principal role. One paragraph earlier, the sharp-eyed reader will note that I declared a ban on any professional theorising here, and though I wouldn't want to inflate this little phrase into anything as grand as a theory, I do confess that it is drawn as much from my work as from my personal experience; it is where I find a fit between the two. Promoting the father who aspires to fail gracefully is not meant to be a counsel of despair; the emphasis is more on the *graceful* than the failing. At work it is something I refer to more with the parents of recalcitrant teenagers than of infants, but I am sure it still applies, and I wish I had realised it more explicitly back then. On occasions at work this throwaway little phrase has raised a much needed smile in desperate times – laughing at life and its comical impossibility – but it also reminds us that our children's successful *leaving* is what we parents work towards; *fledging* is what we call it for birds. If we never failed, there'd be no reason for them ever to leave. And, as if that is not evidence enough, of course there's also encroaching decrepitude – something many a teenage child delights in reminding their parent of; yes, failure is in the job description, along with joy, pride, worry, fury and love.

What follows, therefore, is a series of impressions and thoughts about fatherhood and the finding of my way into this role, gathered around three particular phases; in the expectation of the baby, the arrival, and afterwards.

Expectation

One of the fathers-to-be in our first antenatal classes used to use the phrase 'we are pregnant', or 'our pregnancy', a lot, and I remember reeling in a mixture of horror and delight at the sheer cringeworthiness of his choice of words. At the time I objected piously to the implications in his language; of male appropriation and – almost worse – the assumption that he and his wife were sharing an identical experience. As her belly stretched unfeasibly, and she looked more and more exhausted, while he just got prouder and noisier, this was patently not the case. 'As if he has the faintest inkling of what the full-fat experience of growing another life inside him is really like', I would huff and puff. Fathers, like most humans, are wont to be competitive; perhaps especially so when the rules of the game are broadly unknown. Of course what we were all doing, we fathers-to-be, was trying to work out what to do, how to be, and who to be, and now, just at the point when we'd perhaps begun to rest easy, assuming we'd gathered some clues and competences about ourselves in our pre-paternal lives. Now I look back, I think of the phrase 'pregnant pause', one 'filled with meaning and significance that is yet to be fully revealed', and I suspect that this was indeed our pregnancy, the one we fathers-to-be shared.

It had never previously struck me that nine months is an absolute bare minimum for getting one's life, let alone one's head, ready for fatherhood. It feels daft to admit this, as if I was some hopeless naïf, which perhaps I was, but frankly nobody warned me, or if they did I certainly hadn't been listening. The enormity of the adventure would expand a bit each time I stopped to think about the whole grown-up thing of providing, protecting and securing. Of course there were practical implications such as housing and employment, and these required a level of application beyond the 'later!' that, into my early thirties, had previously worked well enough as a means for prioritising demands. Pregnancy, in contrast, is a startlingly, blindingly, linear thing; it has a beginning, a middle, and an end with a fixed time limit before the obvious new beginning. Up until then, I think time had been broadly circular for me, like a bus route; there'd always be another one along.

Then there was stuff; all the stuff that we suddenly needed. I'd scoffed at the gear friends with babies had allowed themselves to drown in. We resisted the crazier must-haves, and embraced cast-offs from family and friends, but oh, this was still a tide of bright plastic and complicated folding kit that rose and rose, and like King Cnut one could only stand powerless against its advance. A bit embarrassed, I embraced it too, though. The marketers of baby goods are canny, and their siren call is heard nowhere stronger by fathers than in the choosing of prams. I checked wheels and latches with all the attention and excitement that I'd have lavished on a new motorcycle.

Things really ballooned with the arrival of scans and then even more with those first kicks; 'the quickening' to use a lovely old English phrase, to describe the mother's first experience of the baby's movement in her womb.

There was now no avoiding the fact that this was about another, a whole new relationship. It is embarrassing to admit the rather abrupt dawning of my realisation that this new life growing in there was entirely another – 'an other'. This is both a joy, and a terror.

Until the feel of kicks and the sight of a presumed limb drawing shadows across my partner's belly, I think in my own mind the baby had probably been more of an extension to, or a dream by, his mother; or perhaps, in some less definable way, a kind of incremental public broadcasting of the couple, 'us'. But now there was this absolute otherness to contend with, as well. Professionals refer to the 'foetus' in pregnancy, which has always struck me as one of the ugliest imaginable words to apply to what parents think of as their baby. Foetus. Foetid. Stinky. Maybe this language protects workers from feeling too much, or perhaps helps parents to recognise how this separate and independent bundle is not placed here just to satisfy our selfish desires? Do we use this word to stave off too much sentimentalising during a period hedged with uncertainty, and fraught with risk? How many expectant parents have joked with nervous bravado about their little Alien, referencing the film in which something utterly and terrifyingly other bursts forth violently from its startled host? The murky snowstorm ultrasound image (not the startlingly clear images of 21st century obstetrics) that I kept in my wallet did little to dispel this sense of utter mystery, so yes, it was only when I could feel the presence of this otherness with my own hands that I could start out on the new relationship that was coming.

Quickening

In the hot dusk when water congeals
I have sat by pools, loops
Where the river is lazy, watching
For the big fish to rise.
Algae and the reflections of cloud
Hide what is deep and feeding.

At night, now, my spread fingers scan
The surface of your mother's belly.
The skin is taut with presence
But you lie hidden, swimming
In warm waters, rising and falling
With your mother's breath, feeling.

Small ripples on the shiny skin may be
Eddies, just the tickle of waterweed,
A cough, a twitch, giving no sign
Of what grows beneath. But a sudden
Ruck in the smooth film marks a sure
Rise; contact with larger life. Another.

This recognition of a new otherness is where things became more complicated and interesting. As the pregnancy moved on, dim and lazy inklings of recognition coalesced into bright and pressing daylight; how could I have thought this would ever be about just a single new relationship needing accommodation? Instead, now increasingly self-evidently, it involved a whole plurality of new relationships, each one needing renegotiation. Of course there was the mother and baby; of course there was my partner (fast becoming a justly preoccupied mother) and I; then of course there was the baby and I; then all three of us – a new family. But that was just the start of it; there was us and new Grandmother number one; us and Grandmother number two; new grandfathers; new aunts; new uncles, old friends ...

In ways that were both daunting and exciting, fundamental reorganisations started happening right across this network of relationships, without any premeditation or planning, but ineluctably. The image that came to me was one of shifting tectonic plates – a new land mass rising up, forcing existing land masses to shuffle and scrape, move together and apart, in order to make room for the newcomer. In this jockeying for position, everyone's identity has to change a bit (becoming parents, aunts, becoming uncles, grandparents) and in this making of space the friction reveals itself along familiar if forgotten fault-lines. That is a polite way of saying that there were a number of airings of old differences, and renegotiations of boundaries across the wider family; like any tectonic activity, this was accompanied by occasional volcanism, and though fingers were burned, all survived. We survived and managed, but this seemed important, too, not just a reflexive spasm. It marked the fact that things were serious alongside all the excitement and frothicr fcclings. Nothing was quite perfect, and that seemed reassuringly real.

Arrival

The bag was packed, there were some false starts, but the day came. The birth plan was centred on the outcome, not the process; a live, healthy mother and baby, please, and that end justified the means, whatever they might turn out to be. Our observations of other parents had suggested a fairly close association between the level of elaborateness and idealism in their plans, and the level of chaos, distress and disappointment come the messy day.

There had been time to read, and to talk and think about the delivery. I'd delivered babies as a medical student, too, loving the fact that in contrast to so many other parts of the medical training, here one wasn't the awkward bystander, gawping and getting in the way. Medical students had to observe a set number of births, and that meant we would stay, tenacious, for the whole duration of a labour, seeing the midwives check in and out of their shifts, and the obstetricians swooping in at moments of decision or crisis. As a medical student, I felt a rare sense of agency there: I could bring cups of tea, toast, talk, check blood pressures, call for help and offer lots of little practical acts. These last two small words are what, as a father attending the birth of his own children, I so often wanted to offer but felt I couldn't, at least not enough: practical acts. Maybe this is all about narcissism (male, or just my own?) the need to be the heroic fixer, but at the time it just hurt. As a father accompanying the birth one can be beside, behind, with, or around, but never more than that; what you accompany, what is right at the centre of it all, is absolutely not you, and is metaphorically, if not literally, mind-blowing.

First and above all there is the witnessing of great pain in one you love (real pain, not just the hurt of feeling helpless) and the being a bystander to this, and yes, in a blunt and biological sense, the cause, too.

Of course there are warm sponges and cool wipes, and the adjusting of TENS machine settings, and the redirecting of electric fans. There is the negotiating of access to the birthing pool, and the offering of reassurances that it's fine to hate that birthing pool and want the hell out of it, ten minutes after getting in. And of course there is the running into corridors and calling for people, but in the end, the only practical acts any accompanying father really wants to offer are simply and completely out of reach: to take the pain, and the fear of pain, away, and to make everything alright. I remember trying to balance my expressions of empathy with appropriate encouragement, a kind of manly advice, and realising (perhaps, more truthfully, needing reminding) that in this task I had simply run out of lived experience to draw on. Granted, I was a doctor, and had sat with patients, seen things, been right beside suffering, but here this (and I mean no disrespect to my patients) was so different, so viscerally personal, that my fragile sense of competence and agency was swamped. I felt as though the best I could offer was to clown, or channel some blustering coach from best-forgotten days spent in pain and terror on freezing school playing fields; 'come on, you can do it, breathe through the pain, eyes on the prize'. Not much to offer, really.

Next, though, was the kindness and competence of strangers. Being parents-to-be in a maternity ward is like being the next-to-very-smallest of one of those Russian dolls, each figure contained within another, and another, and another. To say we were well looked after by the big NHS mother-doll is hugely to underestimate the many layers and details of containment that we received, from a succession of impressive people who absolutely knew their business. So, as the birth progressed painfully, then falteringly, then stalled, it was made alright to place ourselves in the hands of these people.

The process of birth is immeasurably slow, or was for me; hours of waiting and aching, punctuated with periods when everything is fast and fearful. Everything is heightened, concentrated into the space between four walls; with the small crew around us we might just as well have be on the International Space Station as in a big London hospital.

Our first son got stuck, and was pulled out by Ventouse, a glorified sink plunger. Our second, two years later, got even more stuck, and he was hauled out by Kielland forceps after the obstetrician had been escorted by police, blue-lights flashing, through the middle of the Notting Hill Carnival (the largest street carnival outside Rio) to be there. I can't even now really articulate the fear in those moments, eyes darting from cardiotocograph readout to partner, to her tummy, and back to the eyes of earnest staff, trying to read their poker faces. Our daughter, on advice two years later, was delivered by elective Caesarean section. This was the only delivery that, for me, was relatively free from the pain of sustained helplessness, though not entirely. I still remember the agony of realising that our homemade cassette mixtape ('The Labour Tapes' that had provided musical accompaniment for the arrival of both her brothers), which I had put on as we waited for the procedure to begin, was being eaten by the hospital cassette player. This is, of course a 20th century, not a 21st century, problem, and it seems crazy to focus on such a frittering detail, but that's how it was – everything is heightened, everything suddenly yoked to spooky cosmic significance. These are not ordinary times. As the familiar chords of the opening song on our auspicious music tape started to squelch and gargle I lurched across the room, pushing aside anaesthetist and theatre nurse, to fish out yards of shredded and mangled magnetic tape, shielding the tangle from my partner and blagging all the time nonchalantly 'you know, I think that old tape's got a bit boring' while switching deftly (as I thought) to the radio. Anything to avoid the possibility that this might be interpreted as a sign, an omen, despite the fact that I'm not superstitious. 'You had one job, the music' I could hear a voice in my head saying. Minutes later, our daughter was lifted clear without any of the bruises and dents that her brothers had arrived with, eyes wide open and perfect.

Nothing can prepare you, though you prepare as best you can, and must. All of parenting is like trying out surfing for the first time. No amount of books and conversation with experts can prepare you, and one thing is certain; you must learn the art of falling off and getting back on, and learn it quickly.

As I type, I can feel my prose becoming more impassioned; embarrassing phrases like 'cosmic significance' are appearing. Then again, I can't deny being surprised by this sense of feeling part of something much bigger than me; something like a huge soft engine. It was not that I envisioned us as simple widgets in a giant piece of harsh clockwork, but that we were (and surely remain) in the grip of something both evanescent and yet unimaginably powerful; life, I suppose, and all that is unknowable. When, eventually, I stepped out of the hospital after the birth of our first baby, I discovered that, at the very moment of his birth, on the outside there had indeed been other things going on, cosmic things no less; a lunar eclipse.

Born during an eclipse

A soundless hand of shadow gently delivered
The moon of the full curve in her freckled belly
Just as you were making footfall, slippery
And hot from the dark of your mother's womb.

Hands, heedless of the celestial, helped deliver your mother, too,
Of a ripe mystery which was you
Who'd stretched her belly like a pale plum skin
And now, bright and lazy-eyed, recognised nothing

In the bright air, staring at our eyes, feeding.
In an hour the promiscuous moon was full again,
But not your mother; her waist a soft crescent
With you on it. I'd cut the cord, let loose a new planet.

Next

I hadn't considered the fact that I might be invited to cut the umbilical cord. That this was a ritual as much as a procedure was glaringly obvious, but I'd never really considered it before, even though I must have seen it during my medical student days, and people must have spoken about it. It hadn't registered, though. Perhaps this is unsurprising. It is a hidden ritual, so often carried out in the dark of night (given how many babies seem to arrive in those hours, mine included), with so few onlookers, in the hermetic loneliness of the birthing room. Given how recent the attendance of fathers at births is, we can assume it is also rather a new ritual for fathers, too, but like most strong rituals, there is a powerful ambiguity at the heart of it. There is certainly brutality there;

in the snipping there's a recognition of the sheer toughness of flesh – this is not blancmange you're severing; there is gristle in what links baby to placenta, just as the placenta must shear off, not slip away from the mother. There was a challenge in the invitation to me, too; I am handed steel snippers, heavier and colder than I'd expected, to cut my baby free of the mother. Such powerful symbolism is not readily digestible in the time available to think, and it was over in seconds. In retrospect, I think it hurt just a bit more than it excited me. Like so many aspects of fatherhood to come, it leapt out suddenly and vanished just as quickly, to be replaced by new events. It left me as much with a faint sense of having probably missed the point as it did with the celebration of this new milestone and me still standing. It took me a while to find the words to describe this sense, but in its way, it is familiar even now, and this is OK, because along with the job of failing gracefully there is another job for every parent, which is simply to survive.

Those early hours. Seeing our new son's brown eyes open for the first time, right in front of his mother's face; watching his long, long, and silent gaze into her brown eyes; hearing his mother's gentle and inquisitive 'Hello!'; the tea and toast that someone wonderful and knowing brought and left for us; the quietness, the calm after the storm. Phone calls made from hospital corridors to anxious family. Later, come dawn, a dear colleague working at the same hospital dropped by, filling the room with huge bunches of irises. The first feeds.

With my first new baby now in the world, but staying back in hospital with his mum for checks and the establishment of feeding, I went back home, dazed, amazed. And cried when I was there, suddenly feeling overwhelmed, terribly alone and useless, giddy with exhaustion and fear. Hours later I woke feeling sick, found I had a fever, and heard the unimaginable news of a friend's bereavement, a toddler son lost to sudden infection. Everything was too much. The words of a dear and wise friend whose own baby had been born a year earlier echoed in my head: 'when you have a baby; that is when real fear comes into your life'. At the time, she had said this neither dramatically nor fearfully, but as a matter of plain and simple fact. But so soon? I feared to go in and infect mother and baby, I feared the failure of not being there, I wept, felt woozier and more hopeless, crashing and coughing. The next day or two are genuinely hard to recall, but I do know I felt absolutely terrible – I'm a man who doesn't do being ill very elegantly at the best of times. Notwithstanding the effect of being ill, if fathers can get the baby blues, I certainly had them bad, too.

Of course during this time of my snotty and coughing absence, mother and baby were busy, as they had been through the pregnancy. Feeding was established, and in all the ways that I felt incompetent, they seemed to feel competent; they weren't so much falling in love as getting on and enjoying love, learning each other's ways out here, rather than in there. That much was immediately apparent when, eventually, I was able to drive in to bring them home. It was obvious that the whole umbilical cord business was now from another time entirely; new bonds of recognition and familiarity were already there, building on nine months of an intimacy beyond my imagining. Picking them up from the hospital, I had remembered the right shawl, and the baby grows, and spare nappies, and the car seat. I could do these practical things. By doing and remembering things I could support this new-blossomed love affair that was already obvious between mother and baby, flowering in my absence, unforced, and, from where I stood, easy. What I feared was whether it would ever happen for me, too. Was I forever now relegated to the carrying and the fetching? I was jealous of the looks that passed between them, the adoration, the easy reciprocity, though I struggled to admit this. My head knew this was normal, but beneath the relatively grown up head there is a wild and childish heart.

I may write as if this was all clear to me then, but it wasn't at the time; it was foggy. With my subsequent children's births the same basic pattern replayed itself each time in the early weeks, so it is clearer now in retrospect. I would feel quite exhausted, overwhelmed, and inadequate and worried about whether I could love the new baby. It was a sense that love – or attachment if you want the technical language – was not yet there for me, but that it should be, and worse that this was not enough on my part. I was stalked by a fear of failure because of this, as if doing the practical stuff to support mother and baby – who, if you count the months of pregnancy, were already the best part of a year into their relationship – wasn't enough. As if providing that practical lifting and fetching and carrying wasn't in fact just exactly what I should be doing, not least because it's what I could do. Of course I did this alongside trying to help my partner in the making sense of her own adventure, and this tiny new person's strange ways, but mostly it was the other way round; she showed him to me.

In the case of my second infant son, this self-same worry crept up on me when I'd been busy rebuilding an old fireplace, part of my pragmatic feathering of the family's increasingly crowded nest. I knew that these rather concrete (in this case literally so) efforts were not really what was required.

New

New boy, you come to me so open,
Hurting with the fullness of living.

From the brown eyes your mother gave you
Your smiles and quiet songs burst, a joy

Crystallising, fragile in the dark angry cold.
That I can scuffle, break sticks,

Lay a slow burning fire, and bricks,
Act out the warm holding, hidden

Like a hurt in my own new-born heart,
May you know in this more than I do, of love?

Actually, in all these cases I was just impatient. I'd forgotten that sense, premonition if you prefer, that I'd had in the hospital; the being just a small part of this huge soft engine. In my impatience I'd forgotten that there were other forces at work; forces about which I had little clue, but which surpassed anything my puny head or hands could come up with. My most glaring error – laughable now I look back at it – was to allow room space for the belief that somehow the development of love was something that was up to me to do for my baby. As if my child (or children) didn't have their own parts to play. As if they wouldn't inevitably find their own ways to reach out, take hold of my skittering attention, and gently snare my heart. They reached out and attached to me, of course, not the other way round (or 'Dohh, Dad!' as they might put it now).

Tears

When you were hardly
A thousand tears old
And inconsolable in my arms

You looked up and we
Shared this long moment
Of pure unpremeditated gaze.

In response to my babies' and their mother's promptings, these blue feelings just dissipated gradually over the following weeks, like fog at the arrival of a lazy breeze. There was plenty to do, of course, which helped. What was my role in the months that followed the birth, as everything changed with each new milestone? This is hard to say, not least because there were many sides to me and life was comically, if not cosmically, stretched. This pattern was repeated after each birth; I am reassured to find that we were not alone in finding that just when we wanted to turn inwards and nestle, the demands of the outside world became unnaturally amplified. In the first months after our first child's birth we moved house not once but twice, and I sat my professional exams. In his poem The Second Coming, Yeats wrote poetically of things falling apart, the centre not holding – and at home, with things pulling apart all around us, in typically grandiose fashion I just stretched to cover the holes in the remaining fabric that held us. I'd spend the day at work, early evenings looking for homes on my scooter, come home to hold the baby and give his mother some rest, and snatch hours to revise in the dead of night. My skin erupted in angry complaint, and the nearest we got to lovemaking was my being painted with strong steroids by my partner to calm it down. Since those days I have never needed much sleep, and amidst the exhaustion there was an absolute thrill in all this newness.

Aside from the manic outside activity, there was a thoughtful kind of fathering, too, in which I think I was mostly playing catch up, constantly finding myself left a little behind, caught out by the rising tide of some sudden new developmental shift. I'd realise that I was still stuck in the old rhythm that I'd just mastered, or at other times I'd catch myself going too fast. Then I'd think maybe I was always meant to be just off the beat; musicians call it tempo rubato, stolen time, and it's what adds expression. A new skill, like passing a toy from one hand to the other, a new fascination like the silhouette of a plant's leaves against the window pane was easily missed as I'd go back to the same old papier mâché mobile. But that was alright, as babies like repetition, and anyway their musical mother, whose observation was always more acute, would point out these new time signatures as they emerged.

Of milestones, it was always language – words agglomerating from the soup of babble – that most intrigued me, and the walking that most thrilled. Together, they most marked the differentiation and agency of the individual. Very early in the construction of sentences, words would start getting lined up in quite random ways; worms wriggling on a hook, fishing for father's interest. For a short period I remember my second son went through a phase of asking 'what does [insert random word here] mean?' To be honest, at that time he hardly (it seemed) knew what the question was, let alone making head or tail of the rambling answers that flowed back. What he'd discovered, though, was that this was a good game, guaranteeing a bit of back and forth with Dad, so the hook was reloaded with word after word after word.

What does 'outside' mean?

It is where your mother and I first met,
Though believing ourselves inside at the time.

It is not where you were made.
It is what you were born into,

It is where you will live,
And we are in it together.

In my wilder playful fathering there was adventuring, the finding of new games, dancing, loud music, discoveries of new capacities and strengths. There was a constant recalibration of my understanding of the balance between my babies' terrifying fragility and their essential toughness. Once I had my drowsing son in a kind of over-shoulder hammock device, while peeling potatoes. I had a sense that he loved the random movements as I just got on with things, with him all ensconced, gently bouncing in rhythm with my chores. Things were going well until, as I leaned over the kitchen bin to direct the peelings there, he squirmed and his centre of gravity shifted. I caught him in plenty of time – at least before his head actually disappeared in the bin, and he giggled. I had no fear then, and this was funny, not an occasion for self-mortification but another story about an absent-minded father that was bound in that moment to become a small family legend. The day Dad threw me in the bin.

It isn't all fine and fun, of course. I like to hope that another side to my fathering was recognisable at times, one that was able to attend less to the babies, and more to their mother, tired, ever present, unceasing in her imagination and attention. Of course I am not able to judge this, although I am confident that I failed here as I did often there, with them. Too absorbed in work, self-opinionated, absent-minded, grumpy, grandiose, flighty – all the ordinary stuff. Maybe for parents it is easier to fail gracefully with their child than it is with each other. Grace, as I understand it, is a given thing, not an intrinsic inner quality like temperament, and at the risk of generalising, children are much greater forgivers and forgetters than we adults are. The greatest pleasure in those years of constant change and development was the ability to talk on and on, parent to parent, about what our child said or did today, revelling in the unfurling of a person, and in each other's shared delight. It's this easy relief in shared preoccupations that can make new parents numbingly dull to unchilded friends. Conversely, when a child struggles, the pain that parents feel in failing to make it alright is blinding, and we had our moments when blindly we stumbled over each other.

Perhaps the first steps that I was really proud of in a self-consciously fatherly way were the ones that my children took outwards, away from us; into the world in all its expanse and wideness. Albeit in their earliest years this may have been just the absorption of exploring a toy, and then the first totterings towards the edges of the playground. Fathers, unless I'm alone in this, are inveterate extrapolators and symbol-seekers. In our innate grandiosity and dreaming, we constantly mark things, however messily, with meaning. This is my child; explorer, bold venturer, seer.

Holkham Bay

Naked, not yet four, you stood thigh deep
At the breaking edge of all you knew.

Overlapping slates of North Sea grey
Marched at you from your first utter horizon.

Facing the air and gape of that place,
For seconds you spread your arms wide and,

Just in that brief still confident gaze, held awe.

Then finally there is the laying down of memories. There is something that is infectious for me in my efforts at fathering about creating contexts in which small or even great epiphanies just might take place. Of course an epiphanous moment is by its nature unplanned, and might just as well occur as a child looks out over the bins, or in the school yard, but for me it has always been nature and wildness, so that is where I'd take my children. We worked up from playgrounds to woods and heaths where you could cut sticks and make dens, to sleeping in desolate bothies in wild Scottish mountains, several days' walk from the nearest road. It may be a mark of my children's continued forgiveness that they still indulge me in this now and again, and for that, for them, and for their mother, and her forgiveness, I shall always be grateful.

Chapter 2

The role of fathers in early child development

Kai von Klitzing

In psychoanalytic theories of early development, fathers and triadic relationships play a subordinate role. As we all know, in his first psychoanalysis of a child ('Der Kleine Hans') Freud (1909b) relied exclusively on the reports of the child's father. For him, although the father was the key expert on his child, his role in the process of the developing neurosis was a negative one: he interfered in the love relationship between Hans and his mother by threatening his son with castration and so causing his son's phobic anxieties. In a boy's normal development, an organising role for resolving the Oedipus complex is attributed to the castration complex. On the one hand, Freud (1930a) described the father's protective role, but on the other, prohibition and threat deriving from the father is a fundamental theme in Freud's thinking (Etchegoyen, 2002). In the classic psychoanalytic view, prior to the beginning of the Oedipal drama the father has little importance and the child is mainly influenced by the relationship to the mother, at first as the owner of the nurturing breast, and later as a nurturing and loving person.

But there is also some classical psychoanalytic literature about early triadic relationships and their influence on the child. Klein (1928) stated her conviction that there are early Oedipal tendencies from the end of the first year of life, released 'in consequence of the frustration which the child experiences at weaning' (p. 186). In her view, being deprived of the breast is the fundamental reason why the girl turns from the mother to the father at a very early stage of Oedipal conflict, before penis envy serves to magnify this development later on (p. 193). The recognition of the mother as a good and bad whole object in the depressive position brings an awareness of the separation from the mother object, and enables the infant to recognise other relationships such as with the father. Britton (1989) allocated both a direct and an indirect role in early development to the father; the direct role is that of a figure for identification that supports the child in his/her relationship with the mother, while the indirect role lies in the father's capacity to contain the mother's anxieties and so help her to respond to the infant's needs.

Lacan (1953) considered the third person, the father, to be significant for human life. According to Lacan, this significance is not limited to particular developmental stages. In his view, it is not the real existing father but his symbolic function that represents the essential third element that has to break open the collusion between mother and child. The introduction of the '*nom du père*'/'*non du père*', to be understood as simultaneously the 'Name' and the 'No' of the father, prevents the child from becoming solely the object of the mother's desire. This introduces the child to the world of symbols and language and saves him/her from psychosis (Borens, 1993). Winnicott (1960) dedicated only a few pages in his writing to the father's influence on the child's development and the triangular relationship. According to him, it depends on mothers whether fathers get to know their infant or not. But for the child it is much easier to have two parents – 'one parent can be felt to remain loving while the other is being hated, and this in itself has a stabilizing influence' (p. 115). In Winnicott's view, emotional separation from the mother in the course of development leads the infant to move from a two to a three person relationship. One important function of the father as a third person is to survive the hate the child directs towards him when he has disappointed the child.

Mahler & Gosliner (1955) conceptualised the importance of the father as the third person mainly in the separation/differentiation phase of the second year as a powerful and perhaps essential support against the threat of 're-engulfment of the ego into the whirlpool of the primary undifferentiated symbiotic stage' (p. 210). Abelin, one of Mahler's collaborators, reported that when he organised 'fathers days' in the observational laboratory, he was provided with some 'surprising insights' (Abelin, 1975). He observed that the specific relationship with the father begins in the symbiotic phase and that fathers play a particularly important role in the practising sub phase, standing for distant, 'non-mother' space, for the elated exploration of reality. 'During the course of the separation-individuation process, the father becomes aligned with reality, not yet as a source of constraint and frustration, but rather as a buttress for playful and adaptive mastery' (Abelin, 1971, p. 249). In his theoretical conclusions, he developed the concept of (early) *triangulation* as 'the mechanism that allows the mental organization to pass from the level of relationships (acted, sensori-motor) to images (represented, symbolic)' (p. 233).

So there seems to be a certain move in our developmental thinking from the father as a source of threat and intimidation (at least in children's minds) to the father as the saviour who leads the child away from symbiosis with the mother. There are several levels through which fathers may execute an essential influence on children's development. First, there is the experience of a real father, which depends on whether or not there is a father present in the child's daily life. Second, there is the father as part of the parent-child triad, either in reality or as a concept of the existence of a third person, which opens the experience from an exclusively dyadic relationship towards the experience of a triad and ultimately towards multi-person relationships (Klitzing & Stadelmann, 2011). Etchegoyen (2002) assumed that 'the experience of the father as a "third person" begins to foster the child's awareness of his/her own identity'

(p. 37). In her view and that of many others, this sometimes conflictual but also space-opening function of the father is not exclusively the preserve of the classical Oedipal development of four to six year old children, but is part of a triangulation process, which starts during pregnancy (in the minds of the parents), continues through preschool and school age, and becomes re-actualised in adolescence (Klitzing, Simoni, & Bürgin, 1999). Third, there is what Etchegoyen calls the internal father, which is interwoven with but not solely dependent on the experience of a real father. 'Despite the physical and emotional absence of a real father, there is always some kind of internal picture or representation. Father exists as an object in the internal world' (Etchegoyen, 2002, p. 34). The nature of this internal father can depend on whether or how the child perceives the father directly, but also on how the father is perceived through the eyes of the mother (Marks & Lovestone, 1995).

The real father

In the literature on early child development and parent-child relationships the number of studies involving mothers exceeds the number involving fathers many times over. Nevertheless, since the seminal work of Lamb (1976) there has been increasing evidence that fathers exert an important influence on the early development of their offspring. In a 1977 study, Lamb compared the interaction of 20 infants with their mothers, fathers and an unfamiliar investigator, at home when they were seven, eight, 12 and 13 months of age. Infants showed no preference for either parent in the display of attachment behaviours, but mothers and fathers were consistently differentiated from the unknown investigator. As the children grew older, the children were increasingly likely to direct attachment behaviours to all three adults. Infants responded more positively to father-infant play, mothers held the infants most often to engage in caretaking functions, while fathers held them most often to play. Lamb concluded that father-infant relationships may involve different kinds of experiences for infants than mother-infant relationships, 'such that the two parents have differential influences on personality development from infancy onward' (Lamb, 1977a, p. 167). In the second year of life the infants showed significant preferences for their fathers in the display of attachment and affiliative behaviours. However, fathers were far more active in interaction with sons than with daughters (Lamb, 1977b). In subsequent research it became clear that father involvement varies in different social and cultural settings. For example, Roopnarine, Fouts, Lamb& Lewis-Elligan (2005) examined African American mothers' and fathers' availability, caregiving, and social behaviours towards their infants in and around their homes by comparing 20 lower, 21 middle, and 21 upper socioeconomic families through intensive observations of parents together with their two to four month old infants. Mothers were generally more available to infants than fathers, regardless of socioeconomic status. Mothers fed infants more than fathers did, whereas fathers vocalised more and displayed more affection to infants. In upper socioeconomic families, fathers of daughters were more available than fathers of sons. Both fathers and mothers in the different socioeconomic groups held, displayed affection to, and soothed their infants differently. The authors concluded that, in contrast to European American middle-class families, there might be more convergence than divergence in parenting behaviours of African American parents during early infancy.

Paquette (2004) concluded from a systematic analysis of research on the behaviour of fathers that the different parental roles played by the father are part of a more general function, that of opening the child to the world. In his view, 'men seem to have a tendency to excite, surprise, and momentarily destabilize children; they also tend to encourage children to take risks, while at the same time ensuring the latter's safety and security' (p. 193). Herzog (1998) supported this view, concluding from his observational family studies that in general, each parent plays a distinct role in play with the child. Mothers tend to be homeostatically attuned and to match the child's level of intensity, complexity and affectivity. Fathers tend to be disruptively attuned and their interaction with their child features increased intensity, decreased complexity and increased affective level. Lebovici (1983) pointed to the different experiences of babies when being with a father in contrast to being with a mother. In the relationship with fathers, the young child becomes susceptible to sudden changes and exciting rhythms, and the interaction seems to resemble a lively dance.

Recent research on the neurobiology of human fatherhood has found both similarities and differences in the neurobiology of fathering compared to mothering (Swain, Dayton, Kim, Tolman, & Volling, 2014). For example, neuroimaging studies have found changes in a number of brain regions of human mothers, and similarly in those of new fathers, during the postnatal period (Kim et al., 2010). In a study of 16 fathers the authors found an increase in grey matter (GM) volume in several neural regions involved in parental motivation, including the hypothalamus, amygdala, striatum and lateral prefrontal cortex, but decreases in GM volume of the orbitofrontal cortex, posterior cingulate cortex, and insula from two to four weeks to 12–16 weeks postpartum (Kim et al., 2014). The findings provided evidence for neural plasticity in fathers' brains due to the experience of early fatherhood. In a study on co-parent couples of four to six month-old infants watching own-infant vs. other-infant video clips, Atzil, Hendler, Zagoory-Sharon, Winetraub& Feldman (2012) found that mothers showed stronger amygdala activation and correlations between amygdala response and oxytocin. In contrast, fathers showed greater activation in social-cognitive circuits, which correlated with vasopressin. Swain, Dayton, Kim, Tolman& Volling (2014) commented that these differences might be tied to aspects of differential father behaviour, especially in social play.

In order to examine the co-regulation of positive affect during mother-infant and father-infant interactions, Feldman (2003) videotaped 100 couples and their firstborn child in face-to-face encounters. Parents' and infants' affective states were coded in one-second frames, and synchrony was measured using time-series analysis. Arousal of the infants during mother-infant interactions cycled between medium and low levels, while high positive affect appeared gradually and was embedded within a social episode. By contrast, during father-child play positive arousal was high, sudden, and organised in multiple peaks that appeared more frequently as play progressed. Father-child synchrony was related to the intensity of positive arousal and to father attachment security.

Papousek (1987) demonstrated that intuitive parenting behaviours, e.g. a rich repertoire of adaptive activities toward the baby, originate in humans' evolutionary past and can be observed equally in both mothers and fathers. Schoppe-Sullivan et al. (2014) observed the intuitive parenting behaviours of 182 expectant mothers and fathers in a prenatal play observation using a baby doll and found that fathers' behaviours, although quantitatively less marked than those of mothers, was predictive of fathers' subsequent engagement in developmentally appropriate activities with their babies, but only when expectant mothers demonstrated low levels of parenting behaviour. This finding points to the possible gatekeeping role of the mother, to which Winnicott (1964) has drawn our attention: 'it depends on what mother does about whether father does or does not get to know his baby' (p. 113). In addition, the findings of our research group are that a father's prenatal beliefs about himself as an important relational object for his future baby lead to higher levels of bi-directional activity of the four-month-old baby towards both parents only when the mother was ready to include the father as an important third into a well-balanced triadic play (Klitzing, Simoni, Amsler, & Burgin, 1999).

These findings show that there is a high degree of interdependence between mothers' flexibility (openness towards letting the father be connected to his baby vs. rigid exclusivity in her relationship with the baby) on the one hand, and fathers' readiness to interact with their baby on the other. The father's willingness to be an active relational partner of the infant can play a decisive role in the infant's development when contact to the mother is considerably constrained by the mother's lower emotional availability as a result of her postnatal depression. Field (1998) and many others have convincingly shown that mothers' postnatal depression can lead to depressive affect behaviour in the baby. Babies of depressed mothers are more inhibited and have constrained affects not only towards the mother, but also towards strangers. The babies seem already to have internalised the depressive effects of their mothers. In these risk situations the father can play an important compensatory role. If he is not depressed and spends enough time with his young child, the baby can drop his/her depressive mood when interacting with his/her father, such that trained neutral observers cannot see any differences between the baby's affect expressions and those of babies of non-depressed mothers (Hossain, Field, Gonzalez, Malphurs, & Del Valle, 1994). Furthermore, fathers can play an important role as buffers of the association between depression in mothers and adverse outcomes in infants. In their longitudinal study of 229 women at risk of perinatal depression (in association with their histories of mood or anxiety disorders) and their infants, Goodman, Lusby, Thompson, Newport& Stowe (2014) found that higher levels of maternal depressive symptoms from birth to three months predicted fathers' higher weekday and weekend engagement at infant age three months. Although also showing some indication of an intermittent spill over effect (in the sense that mothers' depressive symptoms can also lead to an increase in fathers' depressive symptoms), paternal involvement at 12 months was also consistent with the compensatory/buffering hypothesis that depression in mothers leads to greater involvement of fathers. However, a large, population-based study of depressive symptoms in mothers (n = 13,351) and fathers (n = 12,884) showed that paternal depression itself can have a specific and persistent detrimental effect over and above the influence of maternal depression on infants' behavioural and emotional development (Ramchandani, Stein, Evans, & O'Connor, 2005). The authors compared the behavioural adjustment of children whose fathers were non-depressed, prenatally depressed, postnatally depressed, or depressed throughout the perinatal period, and found modest support for the psychosocial exposure hypothesis, with higher levels of conduct problems in boys of depressed fathers. They also found that children whose fathers were more chronically depressed had higher overall risks of adverse outcomes. In addition to the direct effects on children's development the associations may also be indirect. For example, depression in fathers in the postnatal period is apparently associated with an increased risk of disharmony in partner relationships (Gutierrez-Galve, Stein, Hanington, Heron, & Ramchandani, 2015; Ramchandani et al., 2008, 2011).

The father as part of the parent infant triad

In psychoanalytic theory it is not the father per se who is attributed an essential role, but rather the father as part of the triad and his role in regulating triadic processes. Classically this is the case in the Oedipal period, when the child's love and exclusive desire towards one parent drives him/her into conflict with the other parent either in the interpersonal dynamic and/or in his/her inner world. The child is confronted with his/her own wishes, the wishes of his/her parents, and with the intimate relationship of the parental couple. But some classical psychoanalytic theories as well as newer empirical research have demonstrated that the experience of triadic relationships strongly influences child development from the outset, and Oedipality signifies only a conflictual culmination point of triadic developmental moves which exist from the beginning of the child's life (Klitzing, Simoni, & Bürgin, 1999).

This view has been taken up by contemporary psychoanalysts in order to conceptualise the influence of triadic experiences on the development of the child's mental functioning. Davids (2002), for example, has stated that the father has to accept the central nurturing relationship of the infant with his/her mother and serves 'as a repository for the infant's experience of the "bad", depriving mother, and this allows the infant to consolidate its relationship with the good object, which is essential for psychic growth' (p. 85). Only with increasing access to the depressive position does the infant's need for splitting and projective identification lessen, and the infant can then become aware of the real qualities of both parents and develop a more differentiated relationship to both mother and father.

In a similar way, Target & Fonagy (2002) criticised earlier psychoanalytic views of a specific role of fathers contrasting with that of mothers in order for the infant to solve the symbiotic ties with his/her mother and to develop his/her own psychic space. For them the father is just another attachment figure for the infant who can develop independent but influential attachment relationships to both parents during the first 18 months of life. But to conceptualise the father's relationship to the infant in terms of just another attachment figure does not meet the special significance of a father figure for the child's development from the beginning, because it uses a relational concept (and a measure), developed and validated specifically by observing mother-infant dyads, for the father as well. This obscures important differences between the mother and the father position. They particularly consider the significance of the 'third person', 'the child's second object' (p. 60) to help create a representation of the dyadic relationship with the child's first object, similar to the child's perception of the self in the mind of the other. In this theory the presence of a third person helps to open the representational mentalising world for the child, but the developmental lines of the father and mother are seen as complementary for this function.

This contemporary form of object relationship thinking, which is closely linked to attachment theory, does not attribute essential significance to the gender difference between the father and the mother position for early development. In this view sex and gender differences between mothers and fathers do not matter for the infant. Fundamental assumptions of psychoanalytic drive/instinct theory that sexuality (in a broader psychoanalytic sense) plays an essential, albeit mostly unconscious role in parent-child relationships are suspended in this view of infancy. Lebovici (1983) noted that the assumption of instinctual economy and associated representations are essential for the origin of the young child's object relationships. Triadic interaction and internal triangular representations seem to be no more than the sum of several dyadic attachment relationships that develop in parallel. Interestingly, this hypothesis of complementary attachment relationships was discussed in the 2002 published work of Target & Fonagy (2002) without any reference to new empirical findings on triads originated by the Lausanne research group of Elisabeth Fivaz and many others.

Since the 1990s the Fivaz group has intensively developed an important experimental paradigm to systematically observe father-mother-infant triangular interaction, the *Lausanne Trilogue Play* (LTP; Corboz, Forni, & Fivaz, 1989; Corboz Warnery, Fivaz Depeursinge, Bettens, & Favez, 1993), which is theoretically embedded in ethology and system theory. This setting was designed to systematically observe how a family of three handles the triangular system of interactions in play as they move through the four possible configurations:

1 In two-plus-ones, when the infant plays with one parent (infant with mother, or infant with father) while the other is a third party, engaging with the active parent while showing an awareness of the third-party parent's presence;
2 In a three-together, when the infant plays with both parents, sharing his/her attention and affects with both of them;
3 When the infant's role is to be a third party during his/her parents' conversation, by attending to the parents' exchange and regulating his/her emotions when not being paid attention.

This standardised situation not only allows the systematic observation of how the parents coordinate to jointly scaffold the infant's social development, but it also assesses whether, when and how an infant is able to relate to both parents at the same time, in each configuration of a triad (Fivaz-Depeursinge, Cairo, Scaiola, & Favez, 2012; Fivaz-Depeursinge & Corboz-Warnery, 1999). This setting was first established for parents with their three to four month-old infants (parents sitting in front of their baby who is seated in a movable baby chair). In the meantime, adaptions for older children and even for the prenatal period Carneiro, Corboz-Warnery& Fivaz-Depeursinge (2006) have also been developed. The quality of family alliance shown during this interactional task is coded along the dimensions 'participation' (e.g. corporeal positions, visual behaviour etc.), 'organisation' (e.g. appropriate distances according to the play phase), 'focalisation' (co-construction of common play), and 'affect sharing'.

Studies by this group and others (for example Klitzing, Simoni, Amsler, & Burgin, 1999) have shown that three to four month-old infants with 'High Coordination' capacities can already share their attention with their parents; they distribute their gaze more or less equally between them and make rapid back and forth gaze transitions. Furthermore, the infants at this age share their affects with their parents,

> addressing triangular bids to them with affect signals in rapid succession. Triangular bids may be positive signals of pleasure or interest when the child is happy with the ongoing interaction, or he or she may signal the need to change the state of interaction by negative signals of tension, distress or protest. The parents validate these bids. In contrast, in 'Low Coordination' interactions, the frequency of the infant's rapid gaze transitions and of triangular bids decreases, and negative bids dominate.
> (Fivaz-Depeursinge, Cairo, Scaiola, & Favez, 2012, p. 11)

In a longitudinal study, measuring family alliance in standardised versions of the LTP during the fifth month of pregnancy and at three, nine and 18 months after birth (*n* = 38), Favez, Fivaz-Depeursinge, Dickstein, Robertson& Daley (2012) identified three longitudinal trajectories: father-mother-child triads with stable high qualities of family alliances, with stable low qualities of family alliances, and qualities declining from high to low. A stable high alliance was predictive of better outcomes in the children at five years of age, especially for theory of mind abilities. In a study of emerging co-parenting alliances assessed in 113 family homes, McHale, Fivaz-Depeursinge, Dickstein, Robertson& Daley (2008) showed that triangular capacities (operationalised as the frequency of rapid multi-shift gaze transitions between parents during interactions) were stable across different interaction contexts. Infants from families with better co-parental adjustment (assessed using several observational and interview measures) exhibited more advanced triangular capacities.

In our research group on child development and early triadic relationships we have carried out several longitudinal studies on the development of the triad, from representations within the parents before the baby has been born to the real triadic parent-child interactions that can be assessed via objective observations. Here are some findings:

1 In standardised interactional observation (Lausanne Triadic Play; Fivaz-Depeursinge & Corboz-Warnery, 2000), well-differentiated relationships between four month-old babies and their fathers as well as their mothers could be observed. Around half of the babies improved their interactional behaviour when both parents offered them well-balanced interactional prompts in the triadic phase of the play. This triadic interaction can easily be disturbed by latent parental partnership conflicts (Klitzing, Simoni, Amsler, & Burgin, 1999).
2 The quality of parental triadic mental representations (especially parents' triadic capacities, i.e. the capacity during pregnancy to anticipate their own relationship with the baby without excluding the partner from the relationship to the baby) significantly predicted the infants' capacities to interact with both parents in a well-balanced and active way (trilogue capacity) (Klitzing, Simoni, & Bürgin, 1999).
3 Well-balanced triadic relationships in the first year without tendencies to exclude are strong predictors for later family functioning and children's individual developmental qualities, such as the child's narrative capacities at preschool age (Klitzing & Burgin, 2005) or the child's abilities to act prosocially in his/her peer relationships at school (Klitzing & Stadelmann, 2011).

In those families where fathers were absent during the first years of the babies' lives (because of separation or other reasons), the mother's inner father concept was most important to enable the child to enter into a triadic world. In cases in which the triadic relationship had fallen apart and the mothers internally and/or externally demonised or devalued the fathers, it was more difficult for the children to develop a stable self-concept and to enter into well-balanced peer relationships.

We concluded from our research that well-balanced and coordinated early triadic experiences, experiences of infants with both mothers and fathers and with the triadic constellation, are all essential for the mentalisation process in early childhood (Bion, 1962; Fonagy & Target, 2000b). The well-calibrated change between the presence and absence of the nurturing object, between the satisfaction and dissatisfaction of needs, is the driving power that leads the child from the pre-concept of an internal object to the representation of self and object. The experience of growing up in a triadic world (with a mother object, a father object and possibly many others) seems to be very stimulating. In such constellations the child can experience not only the absence of an important relational object, but also the absence (and presence) of one object in the presence of the third object. Experiencing differences between the mother and the father object, between their interactional styles (Herzog, 1980, 1998) and their ways of dealing with the child's needs, enables the child not only to experience him/herself in the mirror of the object, but also to find him/herself in relationship with differing objects.

An awareness of the importance of fathers and triadic processes in development has some implications for the psychoanalytic process in work with patients of all ages. Kernberg (1999) has made the case for using the triangulation concept to understand the psychoanalytic process with adult patients too. The analyst should reflect on his/her role in the dyadic transference and countertransference relationship, but at the same time should see him/herself as the different external object, the (possibly excluded) third party. As we see in the development of children in whom the integration of the third (for example the father who represents an object different from the mother object) supports processes of individuation, symbolisation and mentalisation, in the psychoanalytic process an analyst who is not only sensitive but sometimes alters the rhythm of the relational process, or gives unexpected interpretations from a third (father) position, can open a triadic space and thereby catalyse processes of self-discovery.

The internal father

Green (2004) noted that representations of early relationships are formed by conflating internal processes with external experiences: 'From the first union between the psychic representative emanating from the body and the memory traces of the image of the object, a new entity is created: the object representation' (p. 119). In classical psychoanalytic views it is assumed that the building of the child's representational world shifts from the two-person relationship (infant-mother) in the so-called pre-Oedipal phase of development to the three-person relationship (child-mother-father) in the Oedipal phase. But Green indicates the representational role of the father from the beginning of life, paraphrasing Winnicott's famous sentence 'there is no such thing as a baby' (Winnicott 1960, p. 49) as 'there is no such thing as a mother-infant relationship' (Green 2004, p. 101), stressing the importance of the mother's love to the father when caring for the baby. For Green 'thirdness' is a more fundamental constellation not only in child development but in the psychoanalytic model too:

> If we apply this postulation to the analytic situation, we can consider the unconscious as playing the role of the object, verbalization as its expression in terms of sign, and interpretative thought as the process by which the terms are relate to one another. According to various modes of thought and their relationship to a developmental point of view, different sorts of triadic relationships are recognized, and all belong to thought.
>
> (Green 2004, p. 113)

In his view, thirdness in early intersubjective relationships is created via the 'father in the mother's mind' and not so much by a direct relationship of the pre-Oedipal infant with his/her father.

In contrast, Liebman & Abell (2000) emphasised that the 'powerful dyadic relationship' between father and infant influences the growing representational world of the infant over and above the triadic dynamic of father, mother and infant. For girls as well as boys, the internalisation of the pre-Oedipal father-infant relationship is an important basis for the later, more conflictual Oedipal representations. 'The father who adequately relates to his daughter through appropriately nurturing behaviour will be internalized as a benign, realistic, and whole object' (p. 95), which is a crucial precursor to her later eroticised involvement with him during the Oedipal period (Spieler, 1984). For boys it is especially important that destructive (pederastic and filicidal) impulses stemming from the Oedipal drama are transformed into the rough-and-tumble modulated play during infancy (Ross, 1979). The father who is loved and needed in an unconflicted way is assumed to be an important basis for all further developmental transitions, for example to the Oedipal period and to later adolescence.

Bion (1962) referred to the pre-concepts, a state of expectation, of the breast and the penis in the baby, which become concepts when filled with sensory input. The breast is thought to represent the link between the self and other, whereas the penis is understood to refer to the link between the parents, thus introducing triangularity and feelings of exclusion to the baby's experience. In recent years several authors have argued that this kind of psychoanalytic conceptualisation of early paternal influence and triadic relationships is based on the traditional gender roles and family models (father-mother-child) of bourgeois society and cannot persist in the face of modern diverse family structures and parental models. In order to reconcile psychoanalytic concepts of triangularity with the contemporary diversity of living conditions of children and parents, Davies & Eagle (2013) defined paternal functions as being distinct from the role of the father in the life of the infant. They understand paternal function as a set of four interrelated dimensions:

> a separating function in relation to the early symbiotic relationship between mother and infant; a thinking capacity stimulating function via the introduction of experiences of triangulation and linking; a facilitation of affect regulation and frustration tolerance function; and a safety promoting function.
>
> (Davies & Eagle 2013, p. 579)

Following Target & Fonagy (2002), the authors expressed their belief that most aspects of the paternal functioning do not appear to be gendered, so that mothers, fathers and other persons can execute these functions irrespective of their gender. For example, it might be true that the father is a likely candidate to facilitate the separation from the symbiotic mother, but there would be room for this function to be performed by a range of other actors in the world of mother and infant. Even in the absence of a third person, the mother's intense engagement with a nonhuman 'object', such as her career, could similarly contribute to building a triadic relational capacity in the child. In the authors' view what is needed is a 'non-mother' third in whom (or which) the baby is not primarily libidinally invested and who (or which) can support the infant's ability to tolerate frustration and develop autonomy, rather than specifically a male person, not to mention a father. Nor is the function of promoting safety in the face of aggression towards a primary object necessarily bound to a father object. 'It is a fresh parent – an "other" who is of significance to the child – who needed to enable such (paternal) functioning, not necessarily the father nor a male person' (p. 578).

This way of taking any gender-specific aspect out of the 'paternal function' seems to make the concept more applicable for the varied living conditions of the modern world, such as same-sex parenthood, patchwork families, gender fluid parenting etc. Do we move towards parenthood as a gender-free zone? Has parenthood and especially fatherhood nothing to do with the biological origin of life, nor with male and female characteristic or with sexuality? In my view, the formation of object representations, representations of a mother object and a father object, seems to be far more complex than a mere distinction of a mother space and a non-mother space suggests. Following Green's definition of the origins of object representation, the infant's body and the infant's sensory experiences of the parental bodies cannot be completely left out.

The baby experiences:

1. His/her own body with the psychic representative of the instinct (Trieb).
2. The bodies, attitudes and behaviours of the parents or their substitutes.
3. The differences between the parental figures' bodies, attitudes and behaviours.
4. The relationship between the parental figures.

Of course, the relational constellations in which these experiences occur have become more diverse in Western industrialised societies. Nevertheless, the origins of life still have something to do with sexuality (in reality and or in the phantasies of the parents and the developing child), the parental behaviours are not independent from sexual instincts, and the relationships between the parental figures, and the ways in which these relationships are increasingly represented in the mental life of the child are not free from sexuality either (whether in primitive, more mature, or sublimated form).

Herzog (1998) saw the infants' representations of self with mother, self with father, and self with the parental couple demonstrated by play in the sense of a transitional area. He considered play as an expression of an innate ego capacity, which enables the child to perceive and process from the beginning through the technique of ordering stimulus input in a reversible fashion, e.g. trying out various arrangements of incoming data, arranging and rearranging stimulation at first with but eventually without the assistance of another. He argued that to build flexible representations of the self with another it is important that the child accrues experience both of being matched and of matching.

These experiences are more complex than our thinking, which is often shaped by our gender stereotypes, but are not free from libidinal longing and sexual wishes (or from aggression of course). Freud's notion of bisexuality, according to which each human being is endowed with both masculine and feminine sexual dispositions, opens up a vast range of gender aspects in the first relational experiences of the infant. Therefore the pattern described can be expressed beyond gender stereotypes, for example by a mother exhibiting the more challenging interactive style with her child, whereas a father can be more attuned. Other persons (older siblings, friends, other family members etc.) can also perform mother-like or father-like behaviours. But this does not change the basic pattern of differences attributable to gender-specific attitudes, which play a differentiating role in children's experiences of the self with the other, and therefore have a crucial formative influence on the development of self and object representations. It is also worth noting that interactive experiences do not merely follow a one-way channel. In his systematic observational study Herzog (1998) also identified effects of variations in the child's temperament on paternal play style, and effects of gender on the father. It has become increasingly apparent that little girls are considerably more active in shaping their father's behaviours than their male counterparts. Fathers with a firstborn girl perform less 'kamikaze'-like play style with a second born son. In contrast, fathers with a firstborn son and a second born daughter begin to interact with the daughter just as they played with the son. Herzog concluded that the daughter is teaching her father about the ways of interacting in play that suit her. By comparison, boys seemed to be considerably more compliant with the fathers' play style. The representational worlds of the young child and that of both parents are seemingly closely interwoven and form an intersubjective system. Of course, one could argue that these observations took place in so-called 'intact' families with a female and a male parent performing classical role models and that there is in fact much more diversity in contemporary family structures. In analyses of children from families in which the father was absent from early on Herzog observed a father hunger (Herzog, 1980) in children with 'not good enough father experience'.

Conclusion

It appears that human beings have a kind of pre-concept of a father which is best completed by the existence of rich pre-Oedipal triadic experiences, supporting the building of triadic representations in the child which contribute to flexibility and contentedness of the growing personality and a positive developmental outcome. In spite of all the arbitrariness of modern concepts of parenthood without gender specificity, the building of a rich and flexible representational world in the child from early on is much supported by the actual existence and presence of the father and not simply of a 'non-mother person'.

Chapter 3

'The door in the back of my head'

A father's failure to mourn the deaths of his parents

Angela Joyce

Psychoanalysis has been interested in the phenomenon of failure to mourn the loss of a loved person since before Freud's seminal paper 'Mourning and Melancholia' (Freud, 1914a; May, 2001); but there has been very little written from a psychoanalytic perspective, on the long-term impact of a child losing a parent, or indeed both parents, and its consequences when that person becomes a parent themselves. Even less has been written about this child if he is a boy and then becomes a father. The attachment literature has sought to understand the impact of childhood loss on subsequent parenting (Main and Hesse, Lyons-Ruth, etc.) in relation to the emergence of disorganised attachment in a young child but again this has largely been from the point of view of mothers. Even then the impact of losing one's parent(s) seems to be largely considered from the point of view of its impact on the child of the next generation. There has been little if any attempt to describe the *experience* of becoming a parent when the loss of one's parents by death was central to one's childhood. This chapter is such an attempt. I will focus on a clinical case of a father whose wife was referred when their first baby was four weeks old because she was thought to have post-natal depression (PND). He was invited to attend with his wife and child and the work took an unusual and unexpected turn consequent on the revelation he had lost both his parents before puberty.

First, I will briefly consider what might be the significant factors that enable a child to mourn the death of their parent(s), or not. Erna Furman, a child analyst and close collaborator of Anna Freud, was one of the few psychoanalysts who ventured into this realm. Taking a developmental view (Furman, 1974), she proposed that in order to mourn, a child needed to have attained object constancy, a realistic concept of death and the ability to distinguish reality from fantasy sufficiently to work through the loss. For example, the child would need to be able to differentiate the finality of the parent's death from other reasons for his unavailability, which would include being able to distinguish between their fantasies about the death of the parent (for example; 'I caused them to die because I was so angry with them') and the reality of the death. Furman held the view that even young children could be helped to understand and integrate the reality of death if sufficiently supported, although inevitably defences are brought to bear on unbearable feelings as this process ensues. The point is made that mourning inevitably takes place over a considerable period of time and depends on the developmental age of the child and its state, at the time of the bereavement.

Joyce McDougall (1986) describing her psychoanalytic work with a man whose father died suddenly when he was aged seven years old, emphasises not only the fantasies a child might have about what caused the death of the parent, often feeling guilty and responsible themselves, but essentially the capacity of the surviving parent (or the responsible adults caring for the child) to enable the child to mourn their loss so that it doesn't haunt them in their lives ongoingly.

D. W. Winnicott (1965) shows how an 11-year-old boy's reaction to his father's death is to be understood with reference to earlier traumatic losses. Using the Squiggle technique, Winnicott enabled the boy to work with his unconscious knowledge of events when he was a toddler (and lost his mother for a period of six weeks through her illness), to which his mother added the detail that he had been hospitalised as a very young infant for several weeks. Thus, the trauma of the loss of the father was built on earlier traumata, and this complexity needed to be integrated in order for the boy to work through his reactions to his bereavement. The psychoanalytic theory of *après coup* (i.e. that a later event is both to be understood in the light of an earlier one and also the earlier is reconfigured as a consequence of the later; thus, each event is reconfigured and acquires its specific meaning by the relationship between the two in the mind of the subject; see Freud, 1895), helps us to link different life events so that their potential unconscious meanings emerge.

The referral and first session

Rosie (aged early 30s), was referred for parent-infant psychotherapy following a traumatic birth and very difficult first few weeks with baby Tommy, agitated and screaming all the time. The father, Andrew, was very articulate in describing the details of the birth which had clearly frightened him, even though he stressed the sense of failure *his wife* felt in not fulfilling the ideal of the perfect, natural birth. There was also a subtle sense that the disruption to their life as a couple by becoming parents was part of this ongoing 'trauma'.

While this was being described, baby Tommy had stirred from a peaceful light slumber (in contrast to the description of him being a screamer) and his father had taken him onto his lap where he proceeded to give him his little finger on which to suck. They remained like this for most of the session, also raising the unconscious question as to who was the mother whose body had gestated the baby and was struggling to suckle him? Rosie revealed that she was in fact really angry with Andrew because he 'doesn't do things properly', 'wouldn't listen to what she said', to which Andrew replied that he was 'just trying to help', 'wanting to have an input into things'.

In this first meeting with Rosie, Andrew and five weeks old baby Tommy, there had been much conversation about Rosie's parents, who were visiting. I asked if Andrew's parents were also visiting. He had concurred, and it was only when filling in the demographic form with the basic intake information that the bare facts of his parents' deaths when he was a child, emerged. His father died in an accident when he was five years old and his mother from cancer when he was 11 years old. More details of the story of Andrew's previously unspoken memories of the profound losses of his parents were revealed in the Adult Attachment Interview. The hesitant manner of divulging this information was the first indication that it sat uneasily in Andrew's mind.

To give a flavour of the echoes of these childhood experiences evident in the Adult Attachment Interview (AAI), here are some brief extracts:

Q 17. So, you have just become a dad; how do you, if you were to think about being separated from Tommy, how do you think you would feel about that?

Andrew's reply: 'I think at the moment I'm still starting to get to know him still, I mean it's only six weeks, so it's, it's still ... I think, yeah we're still getting to know each other really. Um, yeah, I mean I've ... yeah as I said last week we thought at one stage that we, that he wasn't going to make it or, the immediate thought was pass my mind and it felt terrible for, I mean yeah, one thought that did pass my mind which I, I, I sort of feel a little bit bad about as well, was, with, with yeah with Rosie and they told us there was problems and all this sort of thing I think um, it, it, and one thought that just rushed through my head, oh well, if he's going to, if he is going to die that it's better that it happened now rather than like six months down the road when we are attached to each other but that was like a very like fleeting, fleeting thought. Um ... yeah I think, I think we are getting to know each other more and more every day but I think that it's still...'.

Q 18. If there's any one thing you've learned from your childhood experiences, what would you say it was?

Andrew's reply: {{transcriber note: nine secs silence}} I guess that um, that you know that people can get through anything really I think, I think that you can. Yeah I think, I totally, one main thing that is, like that happiness is, is, is a state of mind, that you can, that you have got a choice, whether you want to dwell on things and be depressed or be unhappy or whether you move on with life and it's, it's a physical choice that everyone's got and, that ... yeah, that, like pull your socks up sort of thing really, get on with life and be happy, don't sort of dwell on things so much.

Q 19. And, what would you want your son to learn from having been brought up by you?

Andrew's reply: 'Oh, that the thing, it's something that I've taught my wife as well I think, is, is that the same thing I think, that you can bring yourself further and further down if, if, if you dwell on things and you can make, make it really bad that you've got, that he's got a choice on life, if he, he wants to look to the past or if he wants to look to the future and that he can, um decide where he's heading and I have a direction in life to head for a place rather than what he's looking back on to I guess'.

The AAI coder made the following observations on Andrew's AAI:

> Coding category: Ds3: Restricted in feeling
>
> Andrew tends to minimise the pain of the losses of his parents in childhood, moving away quickly from the subject with a positive wrap-up. However, he shows indications of a capacity to think about and reflect from his past experience, for example, (when his mother talked to him about what would happen after she died) 'I remember really closing up when she did, when she mentioned about it because it was sort of, not what I could think about . . .'. And regarding his father's death: 'I don't think we never really got over it because we never like talked through it, really'. From what Andrew says, this is his first real opportunity to talk about and explore his feelings regarding his life and upbringing.

Session after the AAI

The material gathered in the AAI usually permeates the parent-infant psychotherapy over time, but in this case Andrew's communications regarding his parents' deaths had a very powerful effect in the countertransference and presented me as the clinician with a dilemma – which seemed to reflect the defensive wall that Andrew had created around his childhood losses. What place was this material to have in the psychotherapy, which indeed had been instituted as a response to Rosie's PND, not Andrew's unmourned losses?

The AAI left me with a curious combination of feelings: that Andrew's childhood experiences were alive in his mind as though they were ever present; but he also was a survivor, and in a determined way had put these events behind him so that he could get on with his life. These diametrically opposed realities co-existed in his mind. This new developmental step of becoming a father challenged that uneasy equilibrium and it seemed that the AAI questions pointed to the immediacy with which those memories challenged him in the present moment, as if time had stood still.

It emerged quite quickly that my sense of Andrew's defensive wall was also shared by Rosie, and she expressed great interest in what was shut off not only in her husband's mind, but from her as his wife. That the early death of his father meant to him that he had no sense of how to be a father was already currency between this couple, but the fact that actually he'd had a father for his first five years and then lost him somehow had been avoided. Except that Andrew's character defence of never planning because life was too precarious was rooted in this formative experience, and its subsequent repetition in the death of his mother from which he had defensively turned away and thus could not anticipate. He said, 'I always, well not always, I was scared about . . . but not really thought it a possibility.' Despite being very emotionally raw, his defensive capacity to 'survive' was paradoxically an important element of establishing the treatment alliance so that he could develop some basic trust that the clinical work was not going to strip him of his necessary defences.

For the next four or five sessions whenever the family came, Tommy was asleep for most of the time, sometimes in Rosie's arms, or in his chair, or occasionally in his father's arms. This made it possible for these more parent-focused issues to be explored. It meant that there was an uncanny sense that I did not meet Tommy for the first two months of our work, reflecting something of the difficulty these parents had in being a family, two parents and baby together, but also placing the parents' difficulties as central to the work. A representation of Andrew as the incompetent parent threatened to develop, a not-unusual constellation when such anxieties are present in a parental couple, and in a splitting process one party has to hold the difficulties. In one session Tommy unusually became very distressed, the first time that he had been so distressed in a session although his screaming and unmodulated affect had been central to the original referral. Rosie had commented several times on how peaceful he was when they came to see me. In this session I actively intervened to disrupt the characterisation of Andrew as an incompetent father and worked with Andrew and Tommy together in the presence of Rosie. In the middle of this process a sentence spoken by Andrew stood out as being over-determined: he said, 'He said why didn't you help me!', apparently referring to Tommy, but it had echoes of his childhood losses and the absence of help for him as a bereaved and suffering child. I heard it also as referring to himself, now, in the session when he was feeling, in the transference, not helped as I pushed him to cope with his infant son, and by implication his own infantile distress. I was working with the unwelcome sense of helplessness that a crying baby can engender, reminiscent also of Andrew's helplessness as a young boy as first one and then the other parent died.

As time went on Tommy was more awake in the sessions which raised the question of what should be the most urgent focus of the work. I had to make a judgement as to what needed to be addressed in a relatively limited treatment. (Winnicott, 1961). I was alert to the impact of Andrew's manner of coping and his defensive strategies on his functioning now as a father. Rosie's PND was abating and attending to Andrew's defensive restrictions of feelings emerged as a significant factor in his capacity both to be a father and also an effective partner to his wife.

Andrew let me know early on how he dealt with the ever-presentness of his experience of the death of his mother, in a metaphor he used: 'the door at the back of [his] head'. Behind this door he put all the unwanted thoughts and feelings about anything he could not deal with. The problem was that when the door opened he was back in the same place, either at the time of his mother's death, or in any place that he could not deal with. It was a mental space in which the ordinary rules of time had been abolished. History could not be placed in the past, as the process of historicity (Bollas, 2013), that is creating meaning out of lived events, had not been possible, for largely defensive reasons. Andrew had disclosed to me that when Rosie's labour started to go wrong, it wasn't just the ideal natural birth that was lost, but he was faced with the real fear that he might lose his baby and his wife, who had to have an emergency caesarean operation. Rosie was surprised when this was mentioned; she knew about the fear about Tommy and had shared it, but not about herself. Here we can see the operation of the locked door in Andrew's mind. It had opened for a moment and pulled into it by association, the potential loss of 'mother', a new representation of his wife he had now to incorporate into his mind. In addition, aspects of Tommy's care were pulled into this same black hole (e.g. in the fear that his screaming and crying would go on forever in a never-ending way): behind Andrew's 'locked door', there was an 11-year-old boy who never was helped to start or stop crying.

As Tommy settled down, the memories of the early weeks of his life became one of these items (locked away), dealt with by applying a rigid regime of infant care in order to keep the experience of helplessness from returning. This parental couple applied Gina Ford's recommendations in her *The New Contented Little Baby Book* (Ford, 2006), so that Tommy became a baby who could only sleep at set times in his cot at home, hated going out in his pram or buggy, had to have his bath/feed etc. at just the right time. I worked hard with the impact of the rule-bound parents creating a rule-bound baby, linking it also with the meaning and purpose of these processes particularly in Andrew: that he could not bear feeling at a loss and helpless. It was also linked with Rosie's anxieties when there was a change in Tommy's behaviour; for example he was a good sleeper at night and she felt good about that, but when he had several nights of slightly interrupted sleep she felt very bad as his mother. These ordinary and expectable changes in his behaviour threatened a rupture in her defensive processes and great fear that she would return to the early days of helplessness and feeling overwhelmed. So, it was that these two parents, for their own reasons, shared this 'solution' of rigidity that influenced detrimentally the way they were caring for their son.

Rosie and Andrew were very responsive to the work, and the anxieties focused on Tommy and his care began to abate. A greater sense of pleasure came into the sessions, anxieties fading. However, the question of the locked door at the back of Andrew's head remained an issue. I was vexed by questions of whether for the onward good enough development of this family some more work needed to be done around that: should it be within a parent-infant psychotherapy model? Should there be a referral for individual psychotherapy? What was Rosie's place in this? Andrew had told me that he had never spoken to anyone, not even his twin brother, about the deaths of their parents since the day his mother died, and every time I broached or made links with these issues he was immediately struggling with tears. Rosie was sensitive to his pain and very much felt that this 'no-go' area was a difficulty in their marriage. She was keen to keep it in focus; Andrew was rather more doubtful.

My reasons in hindsight for suggesting separate sessions just for Andrew were several. I am sure I was influenced by the suggestion from attachment theory that a parent who has an unresolved loss is likely to develop a disorganised attachment with their baby. For Andrew and for Tommy it seemed important not to pass up this opportunity to achieve some measure of resolution. The sessions were deeply painful and notwithstanding 'the locked door at the back of his head', it seemed that this emotional experience was crucially significant for his own life, as well as that of his wife and baby. And for Rosie it seemed she regarded me as an ally. She was acutely aware that because of this 'no-go' area, she felt that her husband was to some important degree a stranger to her. Andrew was surprised to hear Rosie describe him as 'remote and not involved', and at first tried to dismiss it as meaning that men don't know about babies; it was the woman's domain. He was receptive to my point that he was also afraid that if he allowed himself to be not remote but close to this family he had now created, it meant getting close to his memories of his family life that he had lost when his parents died.

But he was terribly afraid of the impact upon Tommy of the well of emotion he was barely able to control in the sessions. If he was to approach this work, he was determined that Tommy should be protected. All this talk had not exactly been welcomed by him; Andrew felt a lot worse than he had before the referral. And it was clear he was deeply troubled by the idea of opening up that locked door. But he was also deeply committed to being a good father to his son and was troubled by the thought that his difficulty in thinking and talking about the deaths of his parents would adversely affect that possibility. Andrew did not want to be referred for separate individual psychotherapy and we worked with the meaning and impact of a decision to alter the frame of the parent-infant work which would include the sense of Rosie and Tommy being on the outside of this special intimate time Andrew and I would have together. We agreed to meet separately for three sessions and then join together for family sessions every fourth time. The rhythm of this arrangement took place during the spring and early summer months.

First session with Andrew alone

In order to help keep the frame of this part of the work in the domain of parent-infant psychotherapy, I saw Andrew in the same room, sitting on the cushions on the floor and with the baby mat between us. Andrew was ready to talk about his memory of the death of his father and its aftermath some years later, his mother's death, and quickly told me the thoughts, fantasies, questions which emerged, if defended against, from behind the door at the back of his head. He had wondered why his mother had died and if it was because he was too much in need of her support such that he was too much of a burden to her. If he hadn't needed her support because of his Dad's death, then maybe she wouldn't have died; what could he have done to prevent this happening, he wondered. It seemed that despite his more rational knowledge of the circumstances of his parents' deaths, at a more unconscious level he felt responsible and guilty.

Guilt feelings are commonly recognised in psychoanalysis as a major factor in difficulties in mourning the loss of a loved person. Thinking developmentally from this psychoanalytic perspective, we also need to take into account the nature of the child's internal relationship with his (lost) parents, particularly the constellation of psychical processes pertaining to the Oedipus complex. This central concept crystallises the wishes, feelings, anxieties and defences that a child feels towards the parental couple and is seen in psychoanalytic terms as a fundamental juncture in the development of the young child. For a boy to lose his father when he was five years old would present him with major challenges as the Oedipal process would be resolving, usually giving way to the phase of latency where the child's interests in the world outside the family would be increasingly established. The propensity for such a boy to feel that his rivalrous feelings towards his father had led to a triumphant victory, allowing him to have his mother to himself would be large, and would likely involve strong feelings of guilt and remorse as well as the painful feelings of loss of a beloved father.

Listening to Andrew talking about his fears that he was too much of a burden for his mother such that she then developed cancer and died, I wondered whether his more unconscious sense of guilt, that held this sense of responsibility in place, was linked not so much with feeling that he had needed too much support from his mother, but that he had become her focus in contrast to the way a latency boy would usually be, moving away. My hypothesis was that his guilt was related to feeling that because of his father's death he could now be the centre of his mother's world instead of father, and that he was to be punished for it. At a more unconscious level I wondered if he felt his wishes had in fact killed his father. The theme of punishment saturated Andrew's account. He talked about his concern for his mother and how he had wanted to be helpful to her, be her 'little man' so that she could have felt supported now that his father was dead. He very quickly got close to the idea that part of his shock and disbelief that she died too was connected with a sense of punishment for not having supported her well enough.

Inevitably in this work, as in all psychotherapeutic work, the clinician has to make a judgement about the pace of the work and also ensure that its content is determined by the patient. To play with the complexity and contradictions of conscious and unconscious thinking in brief focused work is difficult, and I certainly didn't want to push Andrew faster than he was able to go, nor to make leaps of associations to him that would reinforce his defences against their consideration. I continued to work with how these thoughts and fantasies in his mind had both historical and contemporary relevance to him, as a child then and as a father and husband now. For instance, I made links between his shock at his mother's death and his fears that he would lose Rosie (his wife becoming a mother during her labour) and Tommy, his son, as punishment again (the same crime, the same punishment in the unconscious by association), to which he was receptive. In my mind the link was connected with a fantasy of being punished for his Oedipal triumph when his father died but I did not spell this out.

The idea that he was his mother's 'little man' (i.e. old beyond his years, as well as replacing father) also became linked with his wishes for his baby son. I said that I noticed how important it was for him to feel that Tommy was getting on really well, his development going on apace, as though to be a vulnerable little baby was very worrying for him; that he wanted his baby son to be able to show how strong he was, not one who might be quite easily hurt, like he had been. He acknowledged that if he saw a six-year-old or an eight-year-old now who has lost a parent, he saw them as being quite vulnerable, but at the time (when he was that age) he thought of himself as being quite grown up, even that he could control his own destiny! As he saw it, you've got a choice – you can be weak and allow yourself to crumble under external pressures or you can be strong, and you can fight your way through it. His fear of collapsing if he wasn't so strong was immediately then available, as was the necessity of his defence of pushing things away so that he didn't have to risk collapse. He spontaneously made the link with his relationship to Tommy: 'Maybe that's why I do it with Tommy as well … pushing him to keep achieving, driving forward, not relaxing …'

This material shows how this 'individual' work in the context of parent-infant psychotherapy has several purposes. It is not solely to help this father address the unmourned losses of his childhood, but within this model it has other purposes directly linked to his being Tommy's father and Rosie's husband. Additionally, it is to promote his capacities to be a more available father and husband, and here we see Andrew linking his thoughts about how he is himself, with what he expects of his son: his reflective capacity was developing.

Andrew very quickly, and with Rosie and Tommy's help, began to see that his long-held belief that at five or six years of age he was too young to notice that his father had died or that it held any significance for him, was to be questioned. In train with this he began to allow himself to know that he was significant for Tommy. Rosie would tell him that Tommy looked for him in the evenings if he was not home at his usual time, didn't settle so easily if he had not seen him at the end of the day. If a six-month-old could register and show his feelings about his dad's presence and absence, then in all likelihood a five- or six-year-old would certainly have noticed when his dad died and was absent forever. What did he do with this we wondered, and he remembered something he had never understood: that he had a period of bed wetting after his father was killed; nobody had put it together for him. We might think psychoanalytically that his symptom had multiple meanings unconsciously for Andrew, as his ordinary phallic rivalry with his father had perhaps proved so dangerous. In this setting it wasn't possible to explore this any further, apart from acknowledging that it reflected most probably his visceral response to the loss of his father. He began to have a more sympathetic view of himself as the boy who had lost his dad and to have some pity for himself. Andrew revealed that he had always thought he would die young but now he could feel that he wanted to stay alive to be the father to his boy. He revealed that he had thought that he wanted children to keep his family name alive, and we thought about his buried wish to keep his father alive. As we talked more about his sense of what 'father' carried in a family, he was also able to think about what his father missed out on by being killed when his boys were so young; the sadness and the tragedy of it. This work with the meaning of his father's death was a surprise to him as it seemed it was buried behind the trauma of the loss of his mother.

In my last session with Andrew before the summer break, we returned to the loss of his mother, in the context of his discovering that although he had been looking forward to the freedom of being alone, in fact he missed Rosie and Tommy greatly. We had already stumbled on the idea that this unmourned loss of his parents was a way of secretly keeping them alive in his mind. It was a most poignant, painful session with 'the door at the back of his head' open to the memories of the night before and the day his mother died, of which he had never previously spoken. He said that it was strange because talking about it, he realised that it felt much more recent to him than even Tommy's birth seven months before, even though it was more than twenty years previously, a confirmation of my sense at the AAI, that time had stood still at the moment of the loss of his mother.

The family didn't show up for their first session in September and when I phoned, Rosie knew nothing about the appointment. They didn't show the following week either, but Andrew called to apologise. When we met the following week, Andrew's defences were back in place and it proved impossible to re-establish the contact we had had before. Both parents made it very clear that they felt that things were fine now with Tommy and indeed he seemed so, if somewhat precociously independent. The transferential echoes of my absence and loss over the summer had closed the door at the back of Andrew's mind, and I was left to feel the unanticipated loss instead.

Discussion

This brief account of the interrupted treatment of a father, within the frame of parent-infant psychotherapy, describes Andrew's account of his experience of the deaths of both his parents as it emerged following the traumatic birth of his first child. Following Furman, it is possible to see that although it is very likely he had established sufficient object constancy at the point of his father's death, his sense of the reality of his parents' deaths was heavily influenced by his various fantasies, determined by his unconscious wishes, fears, and defences. He had constructed a conscious defence (the 'door at the back of his head') which served to maintain an unconscious illusion that time did not pass and remained ever-present. The emergence of the memories of his mother's death in the last session before the summer break might be understood as a return of the repressed, under the influence of the meaning in the transference repetition of her loss. It was as if the two events were conflated and time collapsed. The recollections of his father's death equally surprised him, as he saw the repetition of his defence of precocity to deny his vulnerability, in his relationship with his son. The relationship then between these two losses and their meaning in Andrew's mind, can be thought about through the lens of the concept of *après coup*. The father's death became in Andrew's mind the cause of the mother's death linked by his guilt for the former in the light of the latter. Andrew had been helped and supported by his mother following his father's death, but after her death there was no one to help him, as the family who cared for him apparently never mentioned it. The other essential feature that Furman and McDougall mention, appropriate help and support to a child on the loss of a parent, was absent. Inevitably I felt disappointed that this work that had been so painful and poignant came to such an end, although I should not be surprised, as indeed I am not; it is perhaps a tale of the impossibility of mourning in the face of terrible loss.

Chapter 4

Waking daddy up

Restoring a father's place in a borderline personality disorder couple

Alejandra Perez

This chapter focuses on the therapeutic work with a father in parent-infant psychotherapy, as he struggled to find his place as a father to his infant son. Alan, his partner Celia, and their two-and-a-half-month-old son, Oliver, were referred to parent-infant psychotherapy (at the Anna Freud Centre) due to concerns that Celia did not want anybody, apart from herself, to engage with baby. Celia had been diagnosed with borderline personality disorder and postnatal depression, and she experienced a sense of catastrophe whenever she became aware of Oliver's separateness.[1] Alan was in a predicament: when he engaged fully with baby, Celia felt worthless and angry. Struggling with guilt, Alan had become passive, withdrawn, and trapped in an enmeshed relationship with Celia. He had given up his studies and contact with his friends and family, and had relinquished any sense of himself as a father.

Fathers who form part of a couple in which the mother is the primary caregiver, face the challenge of coming second in establishing a relationship with their infant child. The value of fathers to their children, as a different object from mother, has been widely accepted (Barrows, 1999; Davies & Eagle, 2013; Lamb, 2002; Woodhead, 2004). However, many fathers struggle to claim a place with their children when their partners do not actively encourage this relationship (Marks, 2002). This is especially the case for partners of mothers with borderline personality disorder who often reject triangular relationships (Britton, 2004; Fonagy & Target, 2000a). Alan faced these difficulties, which were in turn compounded by his own internal conflicts – namely, a childhood experience of an absent father and unconscious fantasies of a damaging father. For all of these reasons, Alan had renounced his place as a father in the family.

For Oliver, this meant that he was lost in mother's delusion of merger, as Alan couldn't act as a helpful separating third. Oliver was also being deprived of the experience of an object who is different from mother; one with a separate, individual mind. Such deprivation has a profound impact on a child's psychic development, understanding of self and capacity to relate to others (Davids, 2002; Davies & Eagle, 2013; Fonagy & Target, 1995).

Father and infant's forbidden attachment

In the first few sessions, I hardly heard from Alan or saw baby Oliver. Celia often held Oliver tightly, covered up and attached to her in a baby sling throughout the session. When Oliver tried to look around at Alan or me, mother would often pull him back towards her and, after a few unsuccessful efforts, he would seem to give up and withdraw into sleep.

Alan would not intervene and was rather an absent presence in these first sessions. Despite his regular attendance in therapy, it seemed as though he were not there at all, as he lay quiet and motionless among the cushions on the floor. Initially, Alan would not speak unless I spoke to him, and then would only reply that he was tired and felt sleepy. Celia, on the other hand, claimed much of the attention, describing her difficulties and displaying great anxiety, anger, frustration, and fear of not being understood. Both Alan and baby seemed to disappear into the background when mother spoke, as if they were not there.

However, I saw glimpses of Alan's sensitivity and connection with baby from the start. Despite Oliver's restricted position with mother, and the great effort it therefore took to move, baby could at times successfully turn to father. When Celia did not notice, almost as though in secret, Oliver and Alan stole glances at each other. In one instance, Celia needed to rearrange her shirt after breastfeeding Oliver, so she handed him to Alan, who up till then had seemed half-asleep. Alan reacted quickly, without anything being said. He extended his arm with an open hand, took hold of baby's head firmly and gently, and held him face upwards. He looked into Oliver's eyes as baby's body rested along his forearm. It was a strong and warm hold, and Oliver seemed content. Alan looked down at baby, who smiled at him. Alan smiled back, caressing his tummy while Oliver held on to Alan's fingers. He rocked him gently; they seemed in a world of their own. Then Celia finished fixing her shirt and turned to them. Alan quickly handed Oliver back; baby squirmed at the rapid change.

It was evident in such moments that Alan was relinquishing a longed-for relationship with his son. This seemed to be, at least in part, due to the difficulties he faced when Celia noticed their interaction, as she would react with anger and despair. Shouting angrily, she would say that she felt Oliver didn't appreciate any of her efforts and that Alan didn't deserve baby's smiles. She would then embark upon a despairing account of her low moods, how desperate she felt and how unhelpful she found others. In those moments, Celia's perception shifted drastically from an idealised fantasy of knowing Oliver best to a resentful view that all was hopeless. The impact on Alan and Oliver was evident: they both withdrew into themselves, Oliver falling asleep and Alan seeming to disappear into the cushions.

Fathers in BPD couples: conflict and avoidance

Borderline personality disorder (BPD) is a complex and serious mental disorder that creates significant psychological distress, not only to the person suffering it, but also to his or her partner and children (Scheirs & Bok, 2007). Relationships involving people with BPD are often unstable, and the relationship is a major source of conflict for both members of the couple. Fonagy & Target (2000a), rephrasing Winnicott's statement that 'there is no such thing as an infant . . .' (in Winnicott, 1960), assert that, 'there is no such thing as a borderline person, there is only the borderline couple – the borderline person and her object' (Fonagy & Target, 2000a, p. 859). However, the borderline person lacks the psychic space and capacity to adequately perceive the reality of the other. Instead, the other is attributed with rejected parts of the self through projective identification. Violent enactments, provocation and manipulation dominate the relationship (Fonagy & Target, 2000a).

Several studies have shown that women with BPD and their partners experience more conflict in the couple relationship than the general population. Partners of people with BPD experience high levels of distress (Scheirs & Bok, 2007). Women with BPD also report lower marital satisfaction, more demand/withdraw communication problems, more relationship instability, and higher levels of violence (Bouchard, Sabourin, Lussier, & Villeneuve, 2009). When examining psychological factors of the partners of women with BPD, Bouchard and colleagues (2009) found that nearly half (44.1%) of them were diagnosed with a personality disorder. Furthermore, both members of the BPD couple had higher rates of insecure attachment representations. These last two results suggest that choice of partner for a person with BPD is not a random process, and that it is likely motivated by complex negative and unconscious factors.

Studies investigating the types of behaviours and communication patterns used by couples during stressful situations, have found that couples in which the woman had BPD showed significantly more negative dominance behaviours compared to a community sample. Women with BPD were also found to use more criticism and verbal attack behaviours than their partners (De Montigny-Malenfant et al., 2013). These negative communication patterns and behaviours are likely triggered by the high levels of emotion dysregulation that women with BPD experience during stressful conversations (Miano, Grosselli, Roepke, & Dziobek, 2017).

Regarding Alan and Celia's interactions, however, they were at first noticeably lacking in overt conflict; they did not disagree, argue, or even talk much to each other. In the moments when Celia reacted angrily to Alan's interactions with Oliver, Alan quickly retreated. It was evident that he was avoiding conflict with Celia by withdrawing and submitting to her delusion of a merged state with Oliver, at the expense of his place as a father and Oliver's development.

An unreflective family fusion

The first few parent-infant psychotherapy sessions with Alan, Celia and Oliver revealed a complicated picture of the family dynamics. These were characterised by an enmeshed, merged fusion in which mother's mind and anxieties took precedence. The intensity of Celia's anxiety and panicked reactions created an unreflective atmosphere and had an impact on all of us.

Britton (2004) describes the challenge of a relationship with a borderline patient: when one can understand and verbalise the patient's thoughts and feelings, one is experienced as helpful. However, when one conveys having a mind of one's own, with different thoughts, one is experienced as unbearably intrusive. Alan had experienced Celia's violent and panicked reactions when he conveyed a sense of being distinct from her in any way. Celia, like many people with BPD, tended to frantically deny difference and insist on agreement of her views (Bateman, 1998; Rosenfeld, 1987).

While father seemed, at times, to be attuned and to respond sensitively to Oliver, he clearly felt conflicted in doing so. At first, Alan seemed to succumb to all of Celia's views. He spoke of his wish to help Celia, knowing that she had had a painful childhood, and that she currently struggled with depression and with forming and sustaining social relationships.

Despite Alan's intentions of being a source of support for Celia, their relationship did not provide her with her longed-for protection from the outside world. In a recent paper, Fonagy, Luyten, Allison, & Campbell (2017) explain that, for the borderline person, a history of adversity, disorganised attachment patterns and emotion dysregulation, generates communication failures at both an interpersonal level and a wider social level. These communication failures create patterns of interaction that are hard to break, with a lack of mentalisation contributing to further social challenges and emotion dysregulation. Importantly, the borderline person develops an attitude of mistrust in the social environment or 'epistemic mistrust' (Gergely, Egyed, & Kiraly, 2007). This mistrust impacts, and lies at the very centre of, relationship problems.

Celia's view was that she knew Oliver best and, therefore, baby needed to be as close to her as possible. Celia often spoke of the relationship she had with her own mother. Celia claimed that her mother 'knew her mind', so Celia did not have to think about her own feelings or try to relate to others. Crucially, Celia felt that this type of enmeshed relationship had protected her from an unreliable and abusive world, and it was the type of relationship that she was convinced would protect Oliver. However, this was a precariously held belief, no doubt due to a deeper lack of epistemic trust where others could never be truly trusted and she could never be truly protected. Celia felt constantly threatened by any signs of reality that disturbed her delusion of merger.

In therapy, I witnessed Celia's difficulties in accurately identifying Oliver's cues and experience, especially when he was distressed. For example, when Oliver cried, at times she heard his cries as though he was coughing and wondered whether he was getting ill. At other times, she either laughed nervously or seemed not to hear him. There were a couple of instances when Oliver attempted to hug her and she mistakenly thought that he wanted to reach the wall behind her. Celia seemed to struggle with Oliver's distress and need for comfort, and with his separateness, as though it shattered her idealised delusion of merger with him (Perez, 2018).

For Oliver, interactions with his mother were clearly confusing and distressing, adding to his own emotion dysregulation. Mother's constantly preventing him from exploring or engaging with others, and father's withdrawal, combined to form a powerful communication to Oliver that separation was not allowed. Oliver was also struggling to make sense of his feelings of distress, as these were often misunderstood and left uncontained. He was also experiencing a father who quickly became withdrawn at any sign of mother's distress.

Davies & Eagle (2013) describe four dimensions of the term 'paternal function': as a 'separating third'; a facilitator of mental structure and the capacity to think; a facilitator of affect management; and a provider of psychic safety. All of these functions are important for a child's development. However, none of these functions were present in Oliver's family. It is likely that Celia did not experience a paternal function in her childhood. Now, she not only lacked these capacities, but she also rejected them in Alan. Oliver's internal world was likely to be dominated by a primary maternal object that did not allow difference or separation, and an ineffectual paternal object that could not helpfully come between them and provide psychic safety. Oliver was becoming more withdrawn, and beginning to prefer toys and objects to people.

The absent father and the rejected, feared father

Early on, Celia told me that the pregnancy had been unexpected. She and Alan had not been seeing each other for long, but on hearing of the pregnancy, Alan moved quickly into Celia's life, dropping out of university, pulling back from social and family contact, and moving into her flat. He explained that he wanted to be involved in Oliver's life and understood how difficult Celia found being around others. In therapy sessions, Alan's fear of Celia's breakdown was clear. However, there also seemed to be something else behind Alan's passivity: an enormous guilt and self-punishment.

It was important to explore Alan's history to further understand his current difficulties, so, after the first few parent-infant psychotherapy sessions, I held two separate meetings, one with each parent. I used the Adult Attachment Interview (AAI) (George, Kaplan, & Main, 1985) to explore their childhoods, their internal representations of their parents, and their states of mind when thinking about these relationships.

In the interview, Alan initially described his childhood as, 'good, normal, nothing much to say really'. However, a picture of a childhood without much contact with his parents slowly began to emerge. Alan's father worked abroad, so spent most of his time away from home. Alan's elder brother was born with cerebral palsy, and Alan's mother spent much of her time taking care of him. It seemed that Alan's parents had little psychic space to think about him. Alan was sent to boarding school aged seven, and he described enjoying his time there. While at first dismissive and minimising of any emotional difficulties that he might have experienced, Alan began to reflect on how he had wanted to escape his family situation, and how boarding school had allowed him that escape.

We explored the mixed feelings he had towards his brother and mother. On the one hand, he felt extremely guilty that he had been spared both his brother's terrible disability and the responsibility of taking care of him. He felt his mother had sacrificed a great deal to care for his brother. On the other hand, he felt resentful that he was excluded from his mother's attention and, with sadness, wondered what it would have been like had he had more time with her.

During the interview I became aware of Alan's defensive, unthinking stance and of his withdrawal. He said he disliked thinking about his mother's constant preoccupation with his brother; it was something that he wanted to put out of his mind. I suggested to him that he wanted to escape all the pain, anger and confusion he felt when thinking about his childhood, and he agreed. I said that perhaps he was also trying to escape the difficulties he now felt with Celia and Oliver. He nodded. I drew some similarities between the guilt he felt towards his brother and mother, and that which he now felt towards Celia.

When trying to describe his father, there was little he could remember of him from when he was a young child. To the question of why he thought his father behaved the way he did during his childhood, Alan shrugged his shoulders, then, after a thoughtful pause said that perhaps his father felt it was best to leave his mother to care for them while he went to work. At first Alan explained that his father felt that his mother 'knew best what to do', as though his father did not know; as though there was no sense that he also had an important place in the family. However, Alan could not completely make sense of his father's withdrawal, despite knowing that Alan's brother was suffering, and that the care required by his brother resulted in a lack of maternal attention for Alan. It was as though Alan's father had decided it was better to avoid his children than be present for them. Alan was thus deprived of both parents and left confused as to the reason behind his father's absence.

Alan expressed some frustration and tension in his current relationship with his mother, particularly around her insistence on seeing Oliver and her disapproval of Celia. However, when talking about his current relationship with his father, he initially denied any feelings of pain, anger or resentment. He described his father as a calm person, and valued this aspect of his character, saying that it was an important quality to have. However, later in the interview Alan expressed sadness about his lack of contact with him. We explored how Alan had made great efforts to be present in Oliver's life, quitting his job and moving in with Celia, because he wanted to avoid being absent for Oliver in the way that he had experienced his own parents as being. However, in many ways he was repeating the pattern of the absent parent: feeling confused and at a loss as to what to do in his role as father, then becoming withdrawn and mentally absent.

In Celia's AAI interview, she described an early childhood filled with trauma and loss. Her father committed suicide when she was four years old, and one of her uncles was physically abusive to her from early on in her life (Perez, 2018).

Both Alan and Celia had suffered the absence of a father during their childhoods. Celia felt threatened by and rejected others. She accepted Alan as part of a merged family fusion, but rejected him as a father to Oliver, with his own views and his own relationship to the child. Importantly, Celia's mistrust seemed to resonate with Alan's unconscious fear of a damaging father.

When Oliver was five months old, Alan called me to say that Oliver had fallen off the sofa and hit his head. Alan had taken him to A&E, where the doctor told him that Oliver was OK. Alan explained that Oliver's fall had happened on his 'watch'. I could hear Celia in the background, telling Alan to explain the incident to me. Alan's call had the feel of a confession. He was evidently worried and seemed to want my reassurance that Oliver was OK but also seemed to be waiting for some sort of punishment. I said that it sounded as though they had both felt very worried about Oliver being hurt. I said that Alan had reacted quickly in getting help. I added that it sounded like Alan was quite shaken by the incident, by the thought of Oliver being hurt. I said that despite getting the doctor's reassurance that Oliver was OK, this did not feel enough, and they both needed me to know about the incident immediately. Alan said that he felt very guilty; that he had been playing with Oliver when he fell off the sofa. We spoke about his guilt and how he associated interacting with Oliver with damage being done to him.

A few weeks later, in one of our sessions, Alan asked me how he should play with Oliver, as Celia felt that Alan's play was too energetic and made Oliver sleep poorly at night. After exploring this further with both parents, it transpired that Celia wanted Alan to stop playing with Oliver altogether, not just before bedtime, as she wanted Oliver to be quiet and still throughout the day and night. Celia seemed to feel threatened by any liveliness in Oliver, as this, again, confronted her with his separateness and his relationship to Alan. Celia's various attempts to keep Oliver still and half-asleep throughout the day were motivated by both fear and anger. Alan, on the other hand, also seemed to feel that liveliness was threatening, as it awakened his own anger and resentment about the neglect and enmeshment he had experienced in his childhood, and that he now experienced in his relationship with Celia. Alan struggled with an internal father who was experienced as benign only when calm and absent, and as uncertain and even threatening when more present. Alan was also evidently struggling with how to express his dissatisfaction in his relationship to Celia and with Celia's relationship to Oliver, as he worried that this would cause a rupture in the couple's relationship, or damage to Oliver. In therapy, we were able to explore how both Alan and Celia had become comfortable with Alan's withdrawn state, and how they both felt threatened by the thought of Alan being a more present father.

Waking daddy up: parent-infant psychotherapy work

Parent-infant psychotherapy work with both parents and baby allows for more opportunities to explore and work on the particular triangular relationships and dynamics in the family – or, in Alan's case, the lack of triangulation. Alan's presence in the sessions, despite his strong tendency to withdraw forced us to think about his place in the family and relation to Oliver, and explore his internal conflicts, in a way that would not have been so easily accessible, or could have been more easily forgotten, had he not been present.

Alan had, up until that point, seemed resigned to Celia's enmeshment with Oliver, and that the family was a kind of fatherless family fusion. Alan was struggling with two different, yet interconnected dilemmas. On the one hand, he couldn't disentangle himself from Celia. Whenever he tried, he was paralysed by her violent verbal attacks or the guilt induced by her depression. On the other hand, he was troubled by his deep resentment towards the mother-baby dyad, which had excluded him in his childhood, and which was now being repeated in Celia and Oliver. His anger and resentment felt too threatening, as it was intermixed with his own unresolved, unconscious guilt of having caused or wished his brother's disability, and now also with a fear of causing Oliver damage. Alan lacked an idea of an effectual father who could successfully act as a separating third without a sense of catastrophe – he lacked the paternal functions of facilitating thinking, and providing emotion regulation and psychic safety (Davies & Eagle, 2013).

An important aspect of the work with the family, then, involved facilitating these paternal functions in each of them and thus creating a triangular space. Developing a therapeutic alliance with parents was crucial, particularly with Celia who often felt misunderstood and threatened to terminate therapy. Meanwhile, Alan, needed to feel it was safe to be separate from Celia's mind, to voice his resentment at feeling excluded and to become a lively, present father.

In therapy, my attempts at understanding each family member's experience had the effect of making them more aware of their separateness. My work with mother indirectly created more space for Alan to interact with Oliver. Alan began wanting more: more time with Oliver; more time to focus on his studies; more time with his extended family. At first, Alan being more present resulted in a period of verbally violent and unreflective arguments with Celia, much like those described in research studies on borderline couples (De Montigny-Malenfant et al., 2013). In relation to Oliver, the more Alan interacted with him, the more his fear and guilt about the possible damage that he might cause Oliver came to the fore. My work with father involved making him aware of his tendency to withdraw, as a defence against this fear, and the impact his withdrawal could have on Oliver.

Of great concern was that Oliver was beginning to show signs of moving into an autistic-like state. By five months, Oliver would often look out of the window during stressful moments in a session, either when mother was describing her distress or when parents were arguing. During one session I noticed Alan look at

Oliver while he was looking out of the window. Oliver had a dazed, absent look on his face as Celia talked anxiously about her ongoing low mood. I leaned over to Oliver and asked him whether he was looking out of the window because he found it very difficult to hear Mummy so upset. I wondered out loud whether he felt that it was all too much and was trying to escape, if only with his eyes and his mind. Alan turned to me and asked, 'Do you think that's what he is doing? I've noticed he does that a lot at home too. At first I thought that he was interested in windows ...' I said to Oliver that I did not think he looked interested in the window, or in anything at all. Instead, he looked rather absent, as though he wished that he was not there. Alan nodded and was deep in thought for a moment. Celia joined in by saying that Oliver often did that. We talked about how difficult it was for Oliver to see Celia upset and to see both parents arguing. By then Alan had sat up, and he asked me what they could do. He was beginning to 'wake up', so to speak, as though he had recognised in himself a similar concern that he had not given voice to. I pointed out that, as soon as we had started to think about Oliver, Oliver had turned back to us, and was now looking at us with interest. As I spoke to Oliver, he smiled and reached out his hand. I touched him, and Celia reached out and held his other hand. He smiled and Celia moved his hand up and down playfully. Alan smiled and commented that he could see the change in Oliver.

A turning point for Alan was becoming aware of Oliver's withdrawal and how it was linked to Celia's enmeshment and his mental absence. Still, he seemed to wait for my direction as he mistrusted himself and as though he were a child himself, needing the guidance and boundaries that his father had not given him, and that he still lacked. He would often withdraw into an absent mental state where he felt that he could avoid causing any damage, and where he became numb to any feelings of concern, doubt or pain. However, when I voiced my concern about Oliver's development, he was confronted with the effect that his absence was having on Oliver. In therapy, he slowly began to feel that, through our exploration, he was more enabled to feel himself to be a parent with his own views and ways of relating to Oliver. He began to feel that his views were valued by Oliver and by me, and that these were increasingly more accepted by Celia. He gradually grew less anxious about interacting with Oliver, and seemed more robust in the face of Celia's panicked and angry reactions. He started to become more confident and more present as a father.

Discussion: an emerging father and an emerging son

Alan's difficulties in claiming a place as a father to his son were due to a combination of challenges: Celia's deep-seated rejection of triangular relationships, and his own unconscious conflict around what being a present father represented.

The challenge Celia presented for Alan was her inability to tolerate him as a separate person coming between her and Oliver, or offering Oliver something different, as she experienced this as a threat to her delusion of merger with baby.

Celia's panic was a strong reminder of her potential to have a breakdown and Alan resorted to a defensive withdrawal. Celia seemed to encourage and feel at ease with an absent Alan, who did not threaten her by confronting her with difference.

The rigidity of defences, lack of mentalising capacity, and lack of emotion regulation in BPD indicate a lack of an internalised paternal function and, most likely, a past childhood with no parent or significant other providing a paternal function. For Celia, not only did she lack a paternal function, she then rejected it in Alan as well.

Celia's violent reactions to difference are familiar to many who have interacted with someone with BPD. There is a tendency either to become provoked into a combative fight, or to end up agreeing with the borderline person's view, thereby relinquishing one's own thoughts and identity.

However, Alan's relinquishment of his identity as a father and relationship with Oliver – which happened all too quickly, and without much of a fight – indicated a deeper, unconscious struggle. Alan's childhood experience of the physical and emotional absence of his father left him with a conscious lack of self-confidence as a parent, but also with a confusing internal paternal object, that was calm and ineffectual at best and damaging at worst. In moments of conflict, Alan resorted to withdrawing mentally, thereby, becoming an absent presence.

As Alan felt increasingly that his place as a father was accepted and encouraged in therapy, he began to interact more with Oliver. This uncovered some of his anger and resentment towards Celia, towards her enmeshment with Oliver, and towards his own mother and brother relationship. This, in turn, exacerbated his fear of becoming a damaging object, and he constantly doubted his interactions with Oliver. Alan manoeuvred himself with great hesitation and sought constant reassurance.

I often pointed out to the parents how Oliver seemed to thrive when he felt freer to explore, to go from father to mother to the toys, and to play with both parents. Although initially wobbly and often tripping up, Oliver slowly became more stable and robust. At one point in the therapy I suggested that we watch a video recording of the previous session, as I wanted to show them Oliver exploring the room and engaging with both parents. They were interested in seeing other sessions too. Mother asked to watch recordings of the first few sessions, when Oliver slept in her arms throughout and she said she felt closer to him. In response to her request, I commented on how aware she was of the separation from Oliver, and how she was beginning to mourn the loss that that entailed.

Alan, on the other hand, wanted to see a recording of a session where he had caught Oliver, preventing his fall. He said that he felt proud that he had done that, and was glad it was 'caught on camera'. We talked about this event and I pointed out that he had caught Oliver not only once, but several times. However, he found it difficult to hold on to the knowledge that he could provide this kind of support for Oliver. Alan had not yet internalised a stable sense of what he could provide, so he wanted my encouragement and to see it again on video. We talked about the guilt that he felt about Oliver falling off the couch 'on his watch' and how he wanted to have an image of himself catching him. I pointed out that it was more than just Alan's physical catching of Oliver that was important. Oliver seemed to have a sense that his father understood his shock, and to be reassured by him that he was fine to keep going. I pointed out how wobbly Oliver had been at first, constantly tripping over and walking into everything in his path; how, at times, he had looked dazed and confused by the world around him. Oliver now seemed more confident in his body and in the room, no doubt due to the change in both parents: Celia allowing him to separate, and Alan being more present.

In the recording that Alan asked to watch, Oliver had, in fact, been walking towards a toy but had tripped over mother's bag, which was on the floor. He lunged forward, his head about to hit the floor. Alan reacted quickly and grabbed Oliver before he fell. He lifted him up and placed him upright again, feet on the floor. Alan had one hand on his tummy and the other holding his waist, as though holding him in place. He exclaimed, 'Whoa little fella!' his voice concerned but calming, his hold firm but gentle. Oliver stood, a bit shaken, and looked at father's face. Alan then smiled and said to him, 'You were about to fall, weren't you?' Oliver smiled back and then turned to walk away. Alan let go and watched him. Oliver went to the toy he was looking for, turned around and looked at father, who smiled and nodded encouragingly. Oliver walked excitedly to the toy and grabbed it, then turned and showed it to all of us, smiling. We all responded by either smiling or clapping. Alan then turned to me and said, 'Did you see that? I caught him!' 'You did', I said, nodding. Both father and son needed encouragement, and were slowly feeling more solid in themselves.

Alan's awareness of Oliver's cut-off state, and of the impact that thinking about him had on the child, had the effect of 'waking' Alan up to his importance as a father to Oliver. Gradually, Alan gained confidence in his presence with Oliver, as if developing a psychic robustness that, in turn, presented Oliver with a strong boundary that he could fall back on, hold on to and push against. The catalyst for Alan had been to feel needed by Oliver, and by me in the work of therapy – needed in a way that acknowledged him as a father. For Alan, his place as a father was something that needed to be restored and encouraged in therapy. It was a role that was unfamiliar to him, not having experienced it in his childhood, and having always had a sense of a father as an ambivalent internal object. This resulted in Alan claiming something of an individual relationship to Oliver. In turn, this change had a strong impact on Oliver, who began to develop in relation to Alan's newfound robustness and engagement with his fatherhood.

Note

1 A fuller, more detailed account of Celia's difficulties as a mother with BPD, her relationship with her baby, and our work in therapy is given elsewhere (Perez, 2018).

Chapter 5

When working therapeutically with a baby's father is not possible

Amanda Jones

Introduction: the problem ...

There are situations when it is not possible to work therapeutically with the mother and father of a baby together. This chapter explores the problem when a psychiatrically diagnosed *serious mental illness* (ICD-10) develops in a woman and when this *illness* can be linked to a woman's relationship with the biological father of their baby. While wherever possible it makes sense to try and offer therapeutic help to the primary parental figures and their baby together, there are times – many times – when a father may not be able or ready to do the arduous emotional work that psychoanalytic psychotherapy requires.

In these difficult situations, a therapist may have to accept that the father's use of powerful (unconscious) defensive processes, especially *splitting, denial, extreme projection* and *omnipotent control*, prevent a therapeutic relationship developing (McWilliams, 2011). A father's actions may communicate that some of his ways of managing emotional complexity through the excessive use of these unconscious defensive processes, will not allow him to become motivated to grow and mature emotionally for the sake of his baby. If a mother is more motivated to try and understand what her illness is communicating about her emotional situation, then it is important to work with her and their baby, even if the father opposes this. Examples of how the above named italicised unconscious defensive processes can operate simultaneously in a father can include: demonising his baby's mother as 'crazy and mental' while considering himself to be free from fault; continuing to be violently forceful towards his baby's mother while stating categorically this behaviour is not happening; refusing to meet the therapist and making false accusations against his baby's mother to social workers and other professionals; believing he is still entitled to have sexual intercourse when this is clearly not consented to; only agreeing to see his baby on his terms; trying to control how his mother treats his baby; trying to charm professionals; completely abandoning the situation and abrogating his responsibilities to his baby. While understanding that a man may consider his continued use of these dynamic and simultaneously occurring defensive processes as essential to his well-being, and so not to be challenged by any professional, for his baby this poses considerable problems and there is no good solution. The perinatal parent-infant therapist needs to calmly, and with compassionate understanding, stand up to the damaging impact these defensive ways of being can have on his baby and on his baby's mother. These situations require careful and ongoing assessment of risk and, to protect the baby/young children and their mother, other agencies such as children's services (child protection social workers), the police and the Family Courts often need to become involved. This adds layers of systemic complexity.

If the father exercises his right to refuse therapeutic treatment, one way forward is to work therapeutically with the mother and baby together to try and help the mother recover from her *serious mental (emotional) illness* and to try and work with her relationship with her baby. This may be all that is possible, and, for her baby, this is essential if a mother is to become able to meet the emotional needs of her baby and, importantly, to meet her own needs more responsibly. This chapter suggests that it is useful to help a mother to come to understand her own use of defensive processes, her partner or ex-partner's use of defensive processes, and the magnetic attraction that drew her to him because of such complex processes. Unless these painful forces of attraction can be questioned and understood, they will be at risk of repeating through the generations. A baby cannot stop this happening. This is the perinatal clinician's responsibility. With time, hopefully, entrenched symptoms of, for example, high anxiety, panic attacks, suicidal hopelessness, violent intrusive images, cravings for mind-numbing substances, deadened numbness and heaviness, nebulous physical pain and inflammation, can recede and even disappear, when a mother comes to understand more fully what may be drawing her towards destructive relationship dynamics. This can then free a mother up to experience her baby differently but, in my experience, it usually involves a painful therapeutic process.

Psychotherapeutic work that cannot involve working with the actual father is complicated in so many ways. One obvious problem writing this chapter is that the actual voices of many fathers I have not been allowed to work with cannot be represented as I would wish: I cannot, like with the mothers, describe the fathers' therapeutic journeys towards becoming more able to consider the needs of their babies. I cannot write about a satisfying therapeutic process of increasing self-awareness and maturing adult parental responsibility in the fathers. I have had to accept that the fathers' use of the defensive processes of *omnipotent control* and *denial* made a thinking therapist a potential threat to be rejected and denigrated, the very same experiences the mothers endured albeit in much more painful ways. Given clear 'No Entry!' commands from the fathers, I had to think about how I could help the mothers and their babies. This chapter is about themes I have come to understand from working with over forty similar cases. One case is described to illustrate how defensive processes can emerge and be worked with, or not, in the clinical process.

The therapeutic work with each mother involved helping her to think about her *(unconscious) choice* to be in a relationship that continually makes her feel shamed, worthless and unlovable. This choice is, perhaps inevitably, influenced by the complicated ways a woman has come to relate to her relationship with her own parents, the sexual couple who made her. Childhood experiences with parents become, in a way, like *internal parents*. Parents who remain alive in our minds, internalised in complicated, distorted, accurate, mixed ways, such that they continually contribute to our thoughts, feelings, and beliefs. These alive beliefs can contribute to how, as adults, we come to 'choose' our sexual partners. Of concern is when a woman may be drawn, unconsciously and magnetically, to being in daily interactions with uncaring and abusive adult sexual partners, partners who may become the fathers of her babies. A common theme in all the cases I am referring to was that the mothers were unconsciously driven to seek relationships with self-seeking, forceful and controlling men who allegedly behaved in violent and abusive ways towards them. In these men, they found states of mind and behaviours that were familiar and resonant with how they experienced their earlier childhood relationships, especially with their mothers. It is important to note that there was also the added problem of the mothers experiencing their own fathers as absent/ineffective/unreachable. What follows introduces some important issues that the mothers and their babies faced.

If these mothers can access parent-infant psychotherapy, the therapist is likely to meet a profound problem from the baby's point of view: the reality that a baby has been unplanned and unwanted and, for the mother, is experienced as another relationship that enslaves her in a potentially never-ending lifelong relationship. At one level, this is with the mother's own internal parents. At another level, it is due to the baby's right to know about, and potentially have a relationship with, his or her biological father. This is hard in every way. Urges to sever and take control and get rid of certain biological facts can emerge. What does this mean for how a baby comes to 'know' about how he or she was made? But also, it is important to keep in mind that mothers may remain in these unwanted couple relationships for some time once their baby is born and unwanted sex may continue to be part of the problem, especially if a mother is submitting to sexual intercourse with the father of her baby for whom she feels no desire. The resentment that can accrue is at risk of suffusing the mother's care of her baby's naked body and result in repeating cumulative relational trauma for a baby. The therapist needs to be able to think about the reality of what is happening and not defensively avoid talking about such sensitive issues.

The focus of this chapter is on how a mother may come to understand in therapy that she also feels in a lifelong enslavement with her own *internal parents* and this emotional experience is being repeated with her relationship with her baby's father. For her baby, one of the risks is that the mother may then transfer these feelings of being trapped and a slave to her baby. Feeling in these roused unconscious relational dynamics means her own unconscious defensive processes are at risk of being continually activated and these will affect how she interacts with her baby's cries for help and attention/affection. The case material suggests it is important to consider how the relationship with a mother's internal parents can remain powerfully active in her mind and may prevent her feeling able to redefine and assert herself differently in her unhealthy relationship with her baby's father. It is important to think about such problems because it is detrimental for a baby's development if his or her mother becomes seriously emotionally ill during the first two years of a baby's life. If this illness becomes understood as an *illness of transgenerational relational origin*, then a woman's relationships, and unconscious patterns of defending herself while trying to survive relating, becomes the focus of therapeutic attention. In a way, it takes many more than two people to make a baby: a group of ghosts may come to the fore when a pregnant woman or postnatal mother develops serious symptoms of anxiety and hopelessness. This means that the work typically entails working with a group of relationships, and this work takes place in conversation with the mother (with her baby present) as she shares her memories and associations about many significant 'others' especially her parents and her experience of them as a couple, and the father of her current baby. A shared experience for many of these women was a sense that they were not that important to their own father and they felt he was ineffective in relation to protecting them from disturbing projections from their mothers. Given that hostile, helpless and frightening internal relationships dominate the mother's current experience, an added problem for her baby may be that a mother may avoid going out or facing others, isolating herself and her baby. At worst the baby may also be exposed to witnessing their mother being abused by their father. But babies may also find ways of making good of more benign or affirming experiences they do have access to, especially siblings (Hrdy, 2016), as the case will illustrate.

In psychoanalytic parent-infant psychotherapy, the psychoanalytic theories introduced so far – namely, the power of unconscious processes, especially defensive processes, and Sigmund Freud's important idea about what he called *the repetition compulsion* (Freud, 1914a) – are clinically useful (Baradon, 2010). The detail of how these psychoanalytic theories can help a baby in clinical practice will now be explored through the case of baby Ben.

Mother Anna and baby Ben

Mother Anna did not present herself as an emergency when she said to her health visitor that she was not coping with baby Ben. With hindsight, she was at acute risk of an impulsive deadly action, either throwing herself or Ben in front of a car or train, or over her fourth-floor balcony. She said to me recently, 'it nearly happened so many times'. Anna was assessed psychiatrically and diagnosed with obsessive compulsive disorder, generalised anxiety disorder and a severe depressive episode. She started medication. The consultant perinatal psychiatrist understood that the relationship between Anna and her baby was suffering. Anna was discussed at the service's weekly multidisciplinary meeting and it was agreed I would offer Anna and Ben psychotherapy sessions.

Some relevant information of the presenting situation

Anna, like many other women, had never been diagnosed with a psychiatric illness before becoming a mother. Yet she had been ill for a long time, she had just never sought help. She had somehow managed to get by. She had been a competent nurse, supporting her household. She was already the mother of an older daughter and son whom she felt close to. She had separated from their father years before due to his violence. Life had meaning but she was also deeply insecure and self-critical. Anna was used to believing herself to be worthless and used to denigrating herself. One problem was that she could not protect herself from finding partners who would confirm these 'ill' beliefs. Although she finished one relationship in which she was debased, she was drawn to another.

In the first few sessions with Anna and Ben, I witnessed how tense Anna was and how hard she found it to touch Ben. At the beginning of each session, as she lifted Ben out of his buggy, she would say, quietly, 'Monster boy …'. The emotional atmosphere was tense and anxious.

It was hard for Anna to be in the room with me due to her expectation that I would be critical. She let me know that at home she spent most of her time cleaning. Ben would be left alone in his car-seat in the kitchen. I said to Anna that sometimes it could help to film a short interaction and watch it together to try and understand what is going on in the mother-baby relationship (Jones, 2006a, 2006b). Anna agreed to this and she could honestly say she thought it would be hard as it was difficult just being in the same room with Ben.

In my mind, certain theoretical understandings help me. Thinking about this chapter reminded me of the following quotation:

> Projections do not pass like magic through the air. They are subtly conveyed to babies by eye contact, facial expression, tone of voice, holding and handling. Video can reveal some of the details which pass too swiftly to observe. However, video cannot adequately convey the emotional impact which we as therapists receive. Our capacity for emotional attunement to details too fine for conscious thinking contributes to the countertransference which informs our thinking.
>
> (Hopkins, 1994, p. 116 [of 2015 edition])

The following example illustrates how Anna tried to manage her emotions being close to Ben. The words she could say revealed why she felt so ill in his presence.

An example of three minutes of unconscious maternal defensive processes in action

This is what happened – my words are in italics:

'Hey dude . . . monster boy . . .'
[Six-month-old Ben was lying on his back on the floor, kicking vigorously.]
'Hey . . . what's Mummy going to do, hey?'
'Mummy's having crazy thoughts dude . . .'
[I then said to Anna that I would pretend to be Ben . . . I said . . .]
'Tell me about them Mummy . . . What's happening?'
'Mummy gets really scary . . .'
'What gets Mummy scary?'
'Everything, everything . . .'
[Ben vocalised and reached for her scarf, still kicking his legs with pleasure.]
'Do you get scared of me Mummy?'
'Yes . . .'
'What do you get scared of with me?'
'Everything, like if I'm doing anything wrong . . . How I am with him and stuff like that.'
'What . . . you worry that I'm going to hate you?'
[Ben rolled to his left, Anna took hold of his right arm . . .]
'You probably do, you probably do . . . monster man . . .'
[Her facial muscles stiffened, as did her right shoulder.]
[She rolled Ben onto his back, he remained keen to reach for the packet of wet wipes.]
'It must be really hard to look after me if you worry that I hate you . . .'
'Definitely.'
'So, you can't think for a moment that I want to be close to you and talk to you?'
[Ben looked at her, eagerly, with his mouth open to vocalise.]
'Nope, definitely not.'
[Ben grabbed her scarf and vocalised, inviting a response.]
'Perhaps you think I think it's better if you stay away from me, except when I need to be cleaned or fed . . .'
'Pretty much, yes, I don't really play with you or talk to you.'
'Mmm.'
[Anna then said how his siblings can play with Ben. She sat Ben up with the packet of wet wipes while pulling back from him.]
'Perhaps you think I prefer them to you?'
'Yes, they are more fun, definitely. You have more fun with them. Hey . . .'
[Ben now reached for her. She used both hands to prevent him coming closer. The tension grew.]
'Did you used to be able to babble and chat with them Mummy?'

'Mmm, not loads but yes, a bit.'
[Five second pause.]
'You've got a belief Mummy that I don't want you near me, but actually you can tell just by how I'm grabbing you . . .
[Ben pulled himself up, using her body, Anna's tension grew.]
. . . how much I want to be close to you . . .
[Ben put his left hand in his mouth . . . She sat him down, creating distance between them.]
. . . so maybe it's something about you not wanting to be close to me. What do you think?'
[Pause. Ben vocalised with a slight tone of frustration . . . Anna held him away from her. The tension emanating from Ben was of confusion, as if something he could not help showing was being rejected.]
'I don't really know, maybe.'
'I think, just that if you think I hate you, I can't imagine why you'd want to be close to me.'
[Anna picked Ben up and moved him away from her. Ben's face was now tense, like hers. She gave him a brightly coloured monkey.]
'What's this?'
[I then said, to both Ben and his mother, speaking with the tone of a concerned therapist . . .]
'What's the normal thing to want to do if you're in a room with someone you feel hates you?'
[Pause from Anna.]
'You'd just want to pu . . . get the hell out of the situation.'

Some thoughts about the interaction . . .

When I turned the camera off, we sat in silence for a few moments. I asked if we could watch it together, straight away. As we watched, I asked Anna how she had felt. She could describe how her heart rate increased when Ben approached her. She said this happened all the time and that she felt on the edge of panic when she had to touch him. I said how important it was she had let herself say the words, albeit quickly and quietly, 'Monster boy' and then, a little later, under her breath, 'Monster man . . .'. I noticed and pointed out to her how the words 'Monster man . . .' came after she had said she worried about doing anything wrong (fear of punishment) and I had said that maybe she worried Ben hated her. I said to Ben that maybe his mummy felt in the presence of a monster man, not a baby. I said this to Ben because I wanted to show Anna that I was in touch with Ben as a baby, innocent in a sense. She nodded. I said how frightened she felt and that she naturally wanted to escape. When, at the end, I asked (with the voice of therapist, no longer imagining I was Ben), what the normal thing to do was if we felt we were in a room with someone who hated us, she replied: 'You'd just want to pu . . . get the hell out of the situation'. I think she repressed the word *push* due to her fear (lifelong fear) of her own anger and, perhaps, of becoming physically violent in retaliation.

Starting to work with the father/mother/other alive in the mother's mind . . .

In this conversation, we were talking about some of Anna's beliefs about Ben: her expectation he would hate her, her belief that he did not want her, her feeling that he was dangerous. I went on to say to Ben that maybe his mum felt trapped with a life sentence. Anna's next association was to say that Ben looked just like his father. Anna had been reluctant to talk about Ben's father before now, telling me in the first session that the relationship had been over since she was four months pregnant with Ben. When I tried to ask a bit more she had become tense. I had backed off as our therapeutic relationship was still new. But having watched the film, Anna said how she relied on Ben's father's help at the end of every day because she could not cope with bathing Ben, it just felt too much after a day of having to feed him and change his nappy. Only then did I realise that although the relationship was described as 'over', Ben's father was actively present, every day, and always on his terms. Anna said he was critical of her, verbally aggressive to both her and her older son, and sometimes physically aggressive. This information was given in a way that minimised the violence that was happening.

A few sessions later Anna could say to me that these daily encounters with someone she felt had malignant intentions towards her had painful resonances with her childhood when, walking home from school, she said that she would dread seeing her mother and hearing what she experienced as constant criticism. Anna believed her mother's beliefs about her and, importantly, she remembered her father as unable and unwilling to protect her from her mother's projections. This is how the intergenerational transmission of emotional trauma can happen: Anna's mother's beliefs, compounded by her sense that she was not worthy of protection, became part of how she believed herself to be. Anna seemed to have been vulnerable to being unable to protect herself from being drawn to an adult sexual partner who would, for his own complex reasons, need to believe the same denigrating beliefs about her. Now she was projecting into Ben her belief he was denigrating, hostile and dangerous, and she was rejecting him. But she was also unable to protect Ben from her projections, repeating the pattern of her own impotent father. Ben had the added horror of witnessing his father abusing his mother. In time, would Ben grow into a little boy who felt chronically confused about his wants for affection and attention? Perhaps he would be at risk of starting to project into others a belief that the world of relationships was not to be trusted. Anna found thinking about these connections hard but a relief.

From baby Ben's point of view ...

In the filmed interaction, it was clear to me that Ben was not afraid of his mother, he still wanted her, and he was persistent. How come, given what I have already written? It is always important to think of *all* the relationships a baby has access to. I knew Ben had two older siblings who Anna had told me enjoyed him. She even mentioned this while I filmed her. I thought Ben had a complicated mix of being with a tense mother who was besieged with hostile and helpless feelings when with him (and yet never neglected his basic physical needs), but he was also with a brother and sister who took pleasure in him when they were home from school. His siblings were affirming experiences and I think this helped Ben find ways to connect to hope when he persisted in the face of his mother's need to resist and push him away. What I witnessed was not the whole experience.

What was helpful, as we watched the film, was how Anna could bravely try to think about the tension and fear she felt, even if she had been managing to provide protective physical care. The words she spoke in the three minutes of film captured their plight and revealed the beliefs and feelings she could not help herself projecting into Ben. In the early sessions, I came to understand that Anna depended upon the continual use of the following (unconscious) defensive processes:

- *Extreme projection.* When Ben approached her, or when she had to touch him, Anna felt frightened he would attack her. She could not stop herself projecting into him a belief his intentions were as malevolent as she experienced his father's. These projections were not just due to her relationship with Ben's father. During treatment Anna could eventually talk about feeling pushed away and rejected by her mother throughout her childhood. She believed her mother felt hostile towards her and this had led to her withdrawing into herself as a child and hiding her feelings. Moreover, she experienced her father as passively supporting her mother's hostility. Anna came to understand how her parent's recent rejection of her need for help after Ben's birth, combined with Ben's father's hostility, culminated in Ben being experienced as a frightening and rejecting figure whom she needed to get away from.
- *Omnipotent control.* At the point of referral, Anna was compulsively cleaning her flat. She said this was to distract herself from intrusive violent images of harm coming to her and baby Ben. Anna was obsessive about trying to control perceived threat in her environment: she cleaned whenever she could and ruminated on her failings in a compulsive way. Her internal talk was torturous, the words she uttered aloud were sparse. At first Anna could not, and would not, change or challenge the many, many ways she controlled her home environment and Ben. On the other hand, she felt she had no right to have any say, or control, about what Ben's

father did to her. Anna was not aware of how she also controlled Ben's experience in the following way: Ben was not allowed to have his own feelings about her. She had taken over his mind so to speak and she 'knew' his intentions and feelings. This is one of the ways the use of *omnipotent control* can intrude into a baby's forming sense of self.

- *Extreme withdrawal.* When we met, Anna could not even know she had been in, and continued to be in, a relationship with Ben's father that exposed her to ongoing abuse. She withdrew from thinking and from certain feelings. She had become numb and frozen and so she accepted her situation. She felt fear with Ben, she felt nothing when his father was hurting her. Anna was caught in an impossible conundrum. She believed she needed Ben's father's help and indeed she did if she continued to believe Ben *was* his father. The problem with being drawn to punishing figures was compelling and she could not think about this and she could not see how this was repeating her early childhood relationships with her own parents. In a complicated way, this was a repetition of her father's emotional withdrawal from her when she was younger.
- *Denial.* For some time, Anna could not know that her choice of partner rendered her children at risk. She was unable to know her baby and her older children were witnessing their mother being harmed and she could not imagine what this would be like for them. She could tell herself that they were fine. Again, this is how she experienced her own father. Moreover, she was in denial of the impact Ben's father was having on her mental health. At first, she believed she was mentally ill and this was yet another of her deficits.

After we talked about the filmed interaction, Anna described how she felt caught in an impossible situation: she felt obliged to look after the baby she had created with a man she could now know she hated. It was interesting how watching the film made it more possible to name and start to talk about Ben's father. When I asked Anna if she could tell me more about Ben's father, she told me they had met a couple of years ago and that he attracted her because he was charming, and he seemed to accept her older children. Quite quickly he wanted to be looked after materially and moved into her flat. He then started to control her emotional environment by criticising her, and then he started to criticise her older son. He gave up work and became financially dependent on her. Silently Anna accepted this, but her mood became flatter as the months went on. Although Anna minimised the verbal and physical violence that started to happen, she could say she became tired of living with a 'time bomb' in the home and that Ben's father had started to be physically aggressive. It is possible to hypothesise that Ben's father found it helpful to project into Anna any feelings of worthlessness. It sounded as if he denied his own areas of inadequacy by relating to Anna as though she was inadequate. Anna also told me that at the very time Anna was planning, with trepidation and fear, to ask her partner to leave her home and end the relationship, she became pregnant with Ben. She was four months pregnant when her baby's father left the home. Ending the pregnancy had never been an option in her mind. The birth was traumatic and baby Ben was ill for a week. The absence of her parents' help at this critical time revived a feeling of being unimportant and unloved (especially with her mother). Clinical symptoms of depression increased even though she managed the care of her children. She felt hopeless, trapped with her new baby. Her obsessive cleaning escalated, and she started to experience intrusive violent images. She would become transfixed by an image of being smashed into by a car when holding Ben, and other horrifying scenarios. This was all invisible to an outsider. She presented as a competent, albeit tense, attractive woman who knew how to care for a baby. Some curiosity about herself was starting to come alive in Anna.

I was then on leave for two weeks. Anna arrived for the session saying it had been a 'crazy time'. She told me Ben's father had hurt her older daughter. He had hit her for defying him and this had caused a red mark that Anna described trying to help with a cold flannel. Anna said the week before assaulting her daughter Ben's father had also pushed her into a wall and she showed me a photo of her face. It was clear she was minimising what looked like a serious assault. I asked if she had called the police. She looked shocked and said Ben's father said it was 'nothing'. He showed no remorse and blamed Anna and her daughter. She told her parents that her daughter had been hurt and this seemed to fall into deaf ears. I turned to Ben, with my heart pounding, and said that his mummy felt so badly about herself that she felt she deserved to be treated badly but I thought she was upset about what had happened to his sister. I said how frightening it was for babies and children to see grown-ups out of control. I could see Anna nodding and I said to Ben that his mummy and I needed to make a referral to children's services as what had happened was very serious. I then said to Anna that a safeguarding investigation should be started, and we needed the help of a social worker. In ordinary language, I explained my concerns that Ben's father's lack of remorse about what had happened, and the way he denied how what he had done was wrong, preferring to see Anna and her daughter as the cause of the problem, were signs of deep difficulties. Anna said that since her daughter had been hit, she had not let him into the flat and it looked like she felt relieved that I had taken it seriously.

A safeguarding investigation took place, and this process was helpful for her older children, and for Anna. When the social worker interviewed Ben's father, he denied what had happened, but her daughter was clear in her description. At the initial child protection conference, I suggested that Ben's father consider some form of treatment. He refused, and he refused to be referred to a domestic violence programme. The children were subsequently placed on a child protection plan. In the brief meetings that I had with Ben's father, it seemed he was using the defensive processes of *denial, splitting, omnipotent control* and *excessive projection*. He described Anna and her daughter as liars, working hard to take over and control a room full of professionals' minds with his words. He was certainly articulate and plausible.

The next phase of the work was difficult for Anna because her intrusive images started to change into memories of the violence she had accepted from Ben's father both during the relationship and since Ben's birth. Memories of her previous relationship also came in, and memories of her own parents' harsh physical discipline and criticism. Anna started to self-harm, compelled by a voice she heard in her mind, a male whispering voice that told her she was the worst mother in the world. Her growing awareness of what her children had gone through exposed her to painful feelings of guilt and, for some time, she could not stop herself punishing herself by cutting her arms and legs after her children had gone to sleep. She also saw her violence towards her own body as the only way she knew how to express her own anger towards herself, Ben's father, her parents and Ben.

Anna has come to a point now such that she can face Ben's father with the fact that he may need to manage some responsibilities in relation to being a father (carefully arranged contact with his child), while having to let go of his omnipotent claim to have some control over her body and mind. The case is now in the Family Court and Ben's father is having to adhere to the authority of the judicial system. In the author's clinical experience, when a mother has managed to change her defensive processes enough so that she understands herself in more complex and compassionate ways, then she may be able to assert herself more and keep herself and her baby safe. Critically, Anna needed to be able *to feel* appropriate fear and anger towards Ben's father and, as we worked with her un-protective internal parents, she became more able to protect herself and her children. In these complex cases, if this can happen, the mother may no longer fulfil the criteria for a psychiatric *serious mental illness*.

Some thoughts about Ben and his persistence and resilience ...

The question about Ben's persistent and fearless seeking behaviours, both in the filmed interaction described and in the weekly sessions I had with them, requires attention. Ben had been exposed to his father's behaviour, and he had been living with a mother who was tense, frightened, rejecting and helpless. Yet Ben showed no fear in his mother's presence and he was still energetically invested in trying to reach her. He was also quick to use me as a consistently available adult. It is important to underline three factors that I think helped Ben: first, his older siblings. I observed how they were playful and loving with him (albeit annoyed and irritating at times too). His older sister was six when Ben was born, and his presence brought forth a wish to be involved in his care. His brother was also boisterously funny. Second, his siblings paternal step grandmother and grandfather were a protective and appropriately caring couple for all three children. It is always important to think about the wider group of emotionally invested others who are involved with a baby. It remains painful to Anna (and to all the other mothers I referred to) that their own parents could not become invested in emotionally mature and caring ways with their grandchildren, thus leaving the mothers I worked with indelibly bereft. Third, Ben's mother consistently looked after all his bodily needs. This does not diminish the pain of rejection Ben was experiencing but it may have contributed to why he did not give up.

For Ben, what is enough? He is now two and a half years old, and he presents as a little toddler who enjoys being alive. Although he remains somewhat (but not always) cautious about how he seeks physical intimacy with his mother, he can still let her know when he wants and needs it. Importantly, Anna can show a lot of interest in what Ben might be experiencing so, in this way, she is not so controlling and intrusive with her own fixed ideas. In terms of Ben's future, and with the other cases, I have found it important for the parent-infant therapist to help a mother imagine the questions her child may ask about his or her father and imagine, at different times in childhood, how she may respond given the inevitable emotional pain that she will have to care for and help. This is more likely to happen when a mother has been able to question herself and understand more why she was drawn to partners who made her feel unlovable and ashamed.

Concluding thoughts

A contemporary understanding about a worthwhile therapeutic goal in parent-infant interventions is to try and improve a parent's capacity to *mentalise* (to have a rich and complex imagination about what their baby might be experiencing, to be able to imagine how the parent may be contributing to their baby's experience, and to be able to tolerate ambiguity and uncertainty). The unconscious defensive processes of *projection, omnipotent control, splitting* and *denial* all thwart *parental mentalisation*. This is one of the reasons it is clinically important to try and understand what defensive processes parents may be relying upon while managing their own couple relationship and their contributions as parents to their baby. In the moment, if a mother believes her projection (such as 'my baby *is* dangerous'), she is not able to allow her baby to have his or her own experience and curiosity about her baby is defensively shut down. If a father believes his projection that his baby's mother *is* worthless, and he is permitted to abuse her, he is not able to allow his baby to value, need and want their mother. In both these examples, the parent is *denying* their baby's right to have a different perspective, and this is an example of how *denial* and *omnipotent control* can operate simultaneously and unconsciously.

With the help of the case example I showed how a woman can use the therapeutic relationship to create in her mind a *new concerned couple who care about both her and the development of her baby.* Anna and I created new memories of her with her therapist as a couple considering/conceiving her baby from different perspectives. In a way, Anna and I also created new memories of a couple considering/conceiving/perceiving her differently. The therapeutic process often entails helping a mother to understand herself less harshly than her earlier experiences with her own parents, while also supporting her to come to know and share more consciously her darker troubling thoughts and feelings in ways that help her to feel accepted and looked after. The case showed how Anna was then able to relinquish troubling ideas and feelings that, in psychiatric diagnostic language are termed *overvalued* (bordering on delusional). In my experience this is not an easy endeavour and the therapist and baby will have to endure some painful emotional processes due to the mother's own use of unconscious defensive processes.

Two guiding principles informed the ideas in this chapter. First, whatever psychiatric illness a woman is diagnosed with, it is always important to work out the unconscious defensive processes a mother is using because these will inevitably affect her relationship with her baby. Second, unhealthy intimate relationships can make humans emotionally (psychiatrically) ill and a woman will be at risk of becoming ill if she is drawn to adult sexual partners who repeat painful relational patterns she may have experienced with her own biological parents and/or primary caregivers. Gaining insight into such repeating patterns is vital for the baby if a mother is to protect herself in the future. When a woman has been repeatedly shamed and violated by her baby's father, enabling her to feel her own authentic and frightening emotions about him can feel life-threatening, especially if she also faces how she has felt unprotected by her own father in the past. Looking after a mother's suicidal despair and urge for revenge is part of the work if her baby is to be freed from being experienced as a 'father/abuser'. This chapter has explored the need to understand and work with the 'father-projected-into-the-baby's-mind', past and present, in his many forms.

Chapter 6

Paternal orientations and the art of being a father

Joan Raphael-Leff

Introduction

Paternity is a complex entity with significance far beyond fathering a child. This chapter presents a model of different contemporary patterns of paternal practice, and a brief overview of changing ideologies since gendered parenthood became a political issue. I argue that egalitarian societies-in-transition such as our own provide diverse personal options. And that chronologically, changes in parenting paradigms co-occur. Fathers can opt to be more nurturing now that women partake of the abundant opportunities men have traditionally enjoyed: *whether* to express their 'generative agency' in parenting. And if so – *when, where, how and with whom* to have a baby, and the nature of their own *optimal connection* to the child and to the other parent. (Needless to say, the gender pay gap and other inequalities still persist, affecting choices.) Feminist unfurling of maternal subjectivity liberated men to contemplate the meanings of fatherhood. Concurrently, an overdue change is occurring within psychoanalytic theory too. It is my contention that as long as mothers were depicted as *placental* – the 'paternal function' was confined to metaphorical cord-cutting to prevent 'engulfment' by the maternal 'container'.

Charting some of the multiple factors that have contributed to the current trend towards a greater degree of paternal involvement, I stress that given the complexity of parent-child dynamics, we must take note of other constituents in addition to emotional engrossment – beliefs, anxieties, wishes and importantly, paternal intimacy and the range of each father's self-motivated 'time-span' of parental responsibility.

By way of qualitative longitudinal studies beginning in the 1970s, I evolved a model delineating four 'orientations', each manifesting different forms of paternal practice:

- a '*Participator*' father who devotes himself to the baby;
- a '*Renouncer*' who treats baby-care as his partner's domain;
- a '*Reciprocator*' who shares care and 'plays it by ear';
- a '*conflicted*' parent who veers inconsistently between extremes.

Although the model depicts 'pure types', diverse patterns of father-care cluster, with some overlap between categories. Over the years this model has been replicated in large scale studies in various countries. But micro-scenarios of daily family experience are always filtered through macro-social expectancies and obligations. So, the distribution of orientations varies cross-culturally, and also over time. However, models have limitations. They are based on provisional hypotheses which simplify a vastly more complex reality. So similar behaviour can have different roots and the same behaviour has different meanings, since affective interchanges are determined by deeply personal variables.

I postulate that for each father, the 'orientation' as played out stems from his own preconscious beliefs about the needs of infants and their intentions. And precipitated by his particular psycho-history – ways of coping with underlying anxieties and the unconscious threat of potential reactivation through 'contagious resonance'. Furthermore, paternal orientation may change with a subsequent baby due to various factors – most notably, parenting experience that modifies his mental representations and degree of defendedness.

In sum, parenting patterns are multifactorial, informed by cultural imagery and socio-economic circumstances (including state provisions like maternity/paternity leave, antenatal/well-baby clinics, crèches, etc.), as well as internal resources, coping mechanisms and emotional tipping points.

Where freedom of choice prevails, families who do not follow a 'traditional' conjugal pattern, tend to negotiate forms of cooperative or unilateral baby-care. These co-parenting permutations of coupled father's and mother's orientations calibrate the 'emotional climate' of each household, which inevitably forms and informs the infant's inner reality.

Caught between generations

At Tate Britain's Hockney exhibition I overheard two lads in school uniform discussing the painter: *'He must have been very good at "Art"!'* declared one. I propose that similarly, a father who excels must have been 'very good' at childhood. If he retains easy access to the curiosity, raptures, and agonies of the child he once was – his enjoyment and compassion will affirm the baby's feelings.

Like Art, fatherhood is a profoundly personal expression of emotion. And like Art fatherhood expands its borders by challenging existing conceptualisations.

Thus, no longer consigned to proverbial 'breadwinning', today's father may choose to be a sling-toting stay-at-home primary nurturer, a part-time carer; a disavowing, or dismissed father; gay or straight; single, married, divorced or in a civil partnership. One is a solo parent; another shares care but does not reside with the baby's mother; or does but is determinedly 'hands off'. A live-in father may be an emotionally detached, workaholic dad or a highly invested devotee of the freshly minted or blended family, or even several families simultaneously . . .

Whatever the format of its many branches, fathering is rooted in archaic soil of his own parenting. But while one father flourishes by adhering to an internalised version of the previous generation's ideology, another holds painful grievances while a third may stretch his representations to improve upon what he himself received. *We may say that today's 'art' of being a father is highly subjective – each striving to experience and express meaningful emotions in his own authentic way.*

Needless to say, this involves many mistakes and moments of failure and betrayal. If digested, these lead to self-discovery and better engagement. However, when troubled fathers feel compelled to act in ways that violate their own wishes or the child's ordinary expectations, therapy is indicated.

Many men feel caught between two generations. Today's involved fathers countenance objectives unknown to their own forefathers. And in these complex times of rapid change, not only do they diverge significantly from their 20th-century fathers, but their 21st-century kids differ even more. The young 'iGeneration' who from birth have imbibed the ambiance of their carers' fast-transmuting electronic, digital, and teleporting voice, visual and tactile communications – inhabit our accelerating virtual-social reality with greater ease than their elders. Conversely, amplified degrees of freedom allow today's Millennial new fathers (born between post-war 'Baby Boomers' and 'Generation Z') to take part in a range of novel exclusive, temporary or regular childcare experiences with their own biological children, or those of their partner.[1]

The seedbed of parenting

Given this considerable diversity, what could we say *unifies* fathers? And what motivates us parents to do what we do?

I suggest that each person's orientation to parenthood is associated with early acquisition of what I term '*generative identity*'. The caveat is that over the past few decades, the very concept of 'identity' has itself become more fluid. We no longer think of a fixed entity but multiple diffuse and dynamic facets of the self – which are context-dependent and do not always neatly cohere. *Gender 'identity'* is a case in point. Although from birth or before each of us is assigned to either the female or male sex, our internal experience lies on a spectrum which ranges from a strict binary division to various subtle gradations of self-identified gender or even agender.[2]

Freud (1905) saw the most 'burning' issues of childhood as distinction between the sexes and the question: 'where do babies come from?' In his view, once solved, these humanising enigmas of early childhood instigate internalisation of the social order of gender, generation and exogamy.

Numerous observations suggest that before psychosexual distinction sets in, infants identify indiscriminately with the capacities of both sexes, naively feeling free to believe they *can be and do everything*. But around eighteen months, as many child-analysts have noted (e.g. Melanie Klein, Margret Mahler, Judith Kestenberg, Irene Fast) a depressive trend sets in when this uncritical 'over-expansive' view is re-evaluated. I ascribe this disenchantment to increasing mindfulness of sexual distinctions and of childhood pre-potence.

The growing toddler is confronted by various restrictions:

- s/he can be only one specific sex;
- each anatomical sex has distinct reproductive capacities;
- it takes both to make a baby;
- parents have potency and an adult (sexual/baby-making) relationship from which children are excluded.

Coming to terms with these facts of life – not being self-made or able to both impregnate and bear a baby, or to become the opposite sex – involves loss of the heady sense of omnipotence. But, and this is the nub, compensation lies in a promise of eventual potency/power, finding a mate outside the family, with whom to have a baby of one's own.

In my view, this momentous shift cannot be over-estimated. Awareness of his/her own generative potential changes the child from being someone else's creation (or creature) to becoming *a future pro-creator* in her/his own right. Many children continue to yearn for ultimate reproduction, conflating true adulthood with being a parent. Some continue to envy the other sex; others disavow limits. In yet others generative identity takes a further leap – they become *creators* ('good at Art') rather than waiting to procreate. Imaginatively utilising their generative agency by creating babies of the mind, rather than a real infant.

Greenacre (1957) famously stated that a 'love affair with the world' – was the prerequisite to developing great artistic gifts. To my mind, if discovering sexual difference confronts toddlers with what they are not, generative agency enables rediscovery of that exhilarating sense of agency.

Generative identity is seeded within a rich soil of identifications and unconsciously absorbed parental transmissions, and cultural prescriptions that are updated over the years with the accretion of wider experience. We now recognise that normative gender expectations are *constructs* – socially determined ascriptions of so-called feminine or masculine qualities or maternal and paternal roles – and hence retractable. But, in recent decades, the sociocultural backdrop is one of a rapidly accelerating pace of life, vastly influential social media, and sadly, early exposure to pornography and widespread violence. Amazingly, innovations of science and technology have even changed our eternal facts of life! We no longer counter absolute restrictions by imagination alone. Today our wildest fantasies of changing sex or transcending anatomy can be actualised in reality. Technology both alienates and empowers – leaving us feeling omnipotent once more!

Paternal engagement

To Freud, on an individual as on a societal level, Patriarchy is rooted in discovering the role *of the father in reproduction*. An awe-inspiring symbol of potency rather than a nurturing presence. Lacan elaborated this as evidence of an 'other', the father, as object of the mother's desire, hence a third term beyond and pre-existing the mother-baby dyad. But what happens to this paternal metaphor when a child learns that the daddy-person is not mummy's impregnator? That 'baby-seeds' may come from an unknown source rather than a sexual partner; that primal scene conception may have taken place in a laboratory to grant a lone-mother's desire for a baby? The child's unconscious representations are beyond the scope of this chapter but suffice to say theory lags behind the newly altered reality.

Towards the end of his life Freud declared fatherhood an 'advance in civilization', based on 'victory of intellectuality over sensuality' (1939, pp. 113–14) – a *premise* by contrast to direct evidence of connectedness in the cord-conjoined birth. A father must take a leap of faith that the baby is his own (and the advent of DNA tests found a high proportion were not). But while genetic tests can now establish paternity beyond doubt, maternal certitude too, has changed. New reproductive technologies can generate families asexually with anonymous origins (through donated gametes and surrogate 'gestational carriers'). Indeed – a mother's parenting partner may be female, or the paternal role may be taken by a genetically unrelated step- or foster-parent, a mentor, adoptive parent, grandfather or grandmother, maternal brother, sister, uncle or any number of other types of self-appointed social 'father', or indeed, a biological 'alterna-dad' (such as sperm-donors with access rights).[3]

Given considerable 21st-century diversity, what then marks out a 'father'? My take is that whether fatherhood is chromosomal or based on donor sperm; whether economically or legally determined, formal or self-designated, solo or co-parenting, in a same-sex or heterosexual family – the 'Father' concept still implies a conscious act of acceptance. Paternal 'artwork' consists of taking responsibility.

The transition to fatherhood – pregnancy, sex and gender

I have argued so far that due to a multiplicity of psychosocial influences from infancy onward, fathers differ from each other in their orientation to fatherhood. Some digress from their own dads' obsolete ways and/or from the new-fangled fads of their sprogs. Yet another major divergence arises with the decision to procreate. Even the most egalitarian partners begin to differ dramatically from each other once they suspend contraception to create a joint baby. In heterosexual couples, the baby grows or fails to, within *her* body, not his. This distinguishing fact of life has a profound impact. *Childbearing remains one of the very few immutable sex-specific differences* (even lactation has been induced in a male to female transsexual). But we humans have a mental capacity that can override physiognomy. Our responses are dependent on emotional orientations not instinctively predetermined by biology or imprinting. We can use our *imaginations* to bridge gaps, to challenge, to alter and expand generative experience. For instance, lesbian partners may decide to conceive simultaneously or serially, or even swap eggs to increase their genetic connection to the offspring.

In men the transition to paternity is so fundamental that it revitalises loaded issues. Each expectant father's feelings reflect the circumstances surrounding the conception and gestation of *this* particular baby, with intrapsychic roots deeply embedded in personal experience of generative identity.

This long-awaited happening is momentous – finally, his turn has come to prove his virility, to become a revered powerful father, even a Patriarch. But considering fatherhood entails great emotional risks for a man who has not satisfactorily consolidated his own agency.

Unsurprisingly, while 'trying' for a baby, temporary impotence is not uncommon, signalling panic at the idea of usurping the powerful archaic father or anxiety about supplanting a weak one. Likewise, when forthcoming paternity reactivates envy of the awesome maternal body, an expectant father may become actively coercive and controlling of his woman's pregnancy. Irrational feelings prevail and affect the couple's day-to-day interaction.

A man may feel overjoyed at conception, but peeved that his impending fatherhood is widely overlooked in the absence of external markers. (Indeed, GPs report increased visits from expectant fathers, many complaining of nausea, stomach cramps, backaches and other pregnancy-like symptoms.) If an expectant father can allow himself to fantasise, his conceptualisation of the baby growing inside his partner's womb is associated with how he imagines his babbling, waddling, inquisitive yet defenceless baby-self was treated. Fantasies about his own conception, gestation and infancy are coupled with childhood memories and family stories which serve to develop a sense of what he wishes for his baby. But when dwelling on the past signals danger, fear of uncontrolled arousal gives rise to antenatal fortifications. Defences may persist postnatally as many new parents feel susceptible to reactivation of their own implicit infantile experience. This experience I termed 'contagious resonance' occurs through exposure to both the infant's raw emotions, and to primal substances of baby-care (Raphael-Leff, 1991, 1993).

Anxiety and paternity

On an unconscious level the changeover from *descendant to progenitor* involves a transition irrepressibly influenced by generative identity and unresolved conflicts. Open-ended in-depth interviews I conducted with first-time expectant fathers found that many conscious preoccupations centred on meeting the demands of an unknown role, and anxieties about the emotions these demands might arouse. The focus of such concerns sets the tone for parenting practice. For some, self-representation as a potential father features concern about their ability to connect, and anxiety about failing the infant by misreading his/her intentions. Others fear they will *become* their fathers, compelled to repeat their own caregivers' failures rather than learning on the trot. For yet others, the present predominates with persecutory anxieties about finding the pregnant body grotesque or imagining the foetus in situ. Others fear future change, apprehension about being exploited by the baby, or succumbing to 'soppiness'.

Clearly, each father's 'orientation' is influenced by the way happy, sad, traumatic, neglectful or abusive happenings have been digested over the years. Significantly, it is not the *actual* experience with his own carers that guides a man's orientation to paternity, but how he has *processed* the emotional ambiance of his own early care and how that influences what he would now like for his own child. Well digested experience, however traumatic it was, enables him to act as a fully fledged partner embarking on the adventure of fatherhood. To do so he must feel free to *recall* his own infantile passions rather than having to inhibit or re-enact these.

So, the 'art' of being an authentic father involves outgrowing the childhood generative wish for a baby who will love him or one he can overpower. To practice as a loving dad necessitates moving beyond the desire to be a sole cherished 'son' to his wife. But when unresolved past grievances are reactivated, the new baby is often conflated with a younger sibling. Rage at his own mother's duplicitous betrayal may be transposed onto his partner. Similarly, his pregnant woman's closeness to their unborn baby and/or fear of his displacement in the new mother's affections evokes deep-seated jealousy. If he remains unable to link feeling neglected now with his past experience, an atavistic need for exclusive attention drives inordinate demands for unconditional love, which may undermine breastfeeding. Conversely, a fear of childbirth as damaging or a simmering Oedipal complex may render a partner sexually taboo once she becomes a mother, leading even a sex symbol like Elvis to abstinence or affairs. By the same token, an expectant mother's reduced libido may incite her 'jilted' partner to sexual belligerence, even rape. Over a third of intimate partner violence begins during pregnancy, and sadistic or aggressive behaviour against the mother or baby is the main cause of foetal injury, miscarriage or stillbirth. Already during pregnancy the degree and quality of paternal involvement is shaped by the expectant father's unconscious anxieties which inform the way he relates emotionally to the unborn baby and to its female 'container'.

Paternal orientations in the 21st century

Given a choice, each expectant father gravitates towards a paternal orientation that meets his own safety parameters. This is partly determined by his particular experience of being parented and specific resolution of generative issues. In addition, orientation is also influenced by the man's age, occupation, current career status and employment conditions, including parental leave. In addition, the household composition, the interval between children and whether he has a person in whom he can confide, also shape the nature of caregiving.

Personal feelings and conscious ideas about the way he wants to parent converge with non-conscious trans-generational transmissions about what fathers should do. This may prove harmonious but if he deviates too much from what he himself received, it may lead to unexpected anxiety. In addition to familial dynamics and personality organisation, orientation is a function of socio-political trends and state provisions, which in turn reflect current cultural values, social priorities and attitudes towards parents and their babies – the future citizens.[4]

A word of caution before elaborating the paradigm of paternal 'orientations': models are always incomplete – they are approximations awaiting further exploration. Assumptions underpinning this model treat manifest behaviours in early parenting practices as adaptive coping mechanisms. Baby-care rests on beliefs about infants' needs and intentions, coupled with semi-conscious anxiety about what meeting these may reactivate through 'contagious resonance'. Coping may involve distorting or denying some aspects of the new reality in order to maintain a familiar sense of self.

I will focus here on three main orientations, and less on the fourth more chronically disturbed category of 'conflicted' parents. Actively preoccupied with, or absorbed in suppressing, unresolved issues from their own childhoods, the latter tends to fluctuate between orientations as anxiety breaks through their habitual defences. Nonetheless, in this group too, fathers and mothers who can use therapeutic help to process their anxieties may alter their orientation with the next baby.

Participators

As the name implies, an expectant father of this orientation wishes to participate as fully as possible in pregnancy, birth and primary care. Much of his generative identity is invested in procreation, culminating in the excited declaration: *'We are pregnant!'* Shadowing the baby intently, he deems his role as shielding the exquisitely sensitive baby from any encroachments. Extreme Participators veer between excited exuberance and intrusive over-protectiveness. Unconsciously, this is to guard against not only the harsh world, or his careless partner, but also his own unacceptable impulses, disavowed ambivalence or destructive fantasies. Fearful of discovering unwanted truths about himself negativity must be erased, but creeps in under the radar.

Manifestations of Participator behaviours are fed by a variety of differing identifications and anxieties underpinning these. When this stance draws on primary identification with a nurturing mother his emphasis is on communing with the unborn baby, 'nourishing' it with his love and semen. But an expectant Participator who feels frustratedly cheated by the mother-mediated gateway to his child and distrustful of his partner's capacity to grow their baby, requires ongoing external verification of his baby's wellbeing. Conversely, a man who is predominantly identified with the foetus rather than the mother, regards himself as the baby's interpreter (ante and postnatally). His narcissistic investment heightens anxiety about the baby's fragility. S/he may seem trapped inside, or starved of sufficient nutrients, or exposed to noxious input. Unconsciously associating the baby-to-be with his idealised baby-self feeds a fervent wish to champion the child and keep all undesirable experience at bay – by promoting a blissful gestation and 'seamless' transition between womb and world by calm 'natural' childbirth. Unconsciously, the perfect infancy means re-creating the womb in a cosy, bountiful organic environment which he can control.

In love with the amazing newborn safely papoosed in his marsupial sling like an external pregnancy, the father is ecstatic. He participates in all baby-care activities, and believing that the symbiotically connected baby communicates his/her needs through every sound and every twitch, feels he must stay close, even at night, to decipher and fulfil every desire. His own separation anxiety may be a prime motivator of over-involvement.

However, idealised wishes are open to frustration. If the baby requires incubation, or if the mother is equally in love and wishes to breastfeed exclusively or thwarts his need to be full-time main carer, he may feel devastated, experiencing terrible perinatal sadness and guilt at having already let the baby down.

Renouncers

By contrast, fathers in this category are embedded in a male/female divide that regards childbearing, birth and nurturing as the province of women. Nonetheless, the pregnancy is proof of his virility ('Pretty big bump, huh?!').

On a deeper level what impels this orientation is anxiety about becoming overwhelmed by implacable emotion – the baby's or his own (regarded as 'unmanly' – feminine and/or infantile). His coping mechanisms include dissociation, withdrawal, and splitting. These serve to keep him 'cool' and also protect him against the *baby*, to whom, through psychic defence mechanisms of projective identification, he attributes unacceptable dependent, needy or greedy parts of himself. His expressed concern in protecting her during pregnancy is that the 'parasitic' foetus is draining its hostess' resources, decreasing her energy and availability.

Alarmed by his partner's 'moodiness' and tendency towards introspection, he tries to remain calm, emulating an authoritative father figure. Priding himself on his rationality, he unconsciously fears being 'taken over' by the baby, falling in love and making a fool of himself. So, already during the pregnancy, schooled in emotional restraint this expectant father will fortify his 'masculine' attributes to prevent any gush of sentiment breaking through. Driven by caution he states that his interest in the foetus is 'purely intellectual', safeguarding himself against the risk of 'losing it' by treating pregnancy as uncertain and labour as a medical event to be managed by experts. He resists becoming attached to the unborn baby in case anything goes wrong. Dreading exposure to high emotions, he plans to avoid the birth by promoting a project of his own to coincide with it. If compelled to be there he ensures technological interventions (epidural, monitors, elective C-section) to mitigate the pain and gore, and to control intense feelings surrounding birth.

While proud of becoming a father, the Renouncer father does not anticipate being involved much until the child 'can talk or play football'; he sees his role as limit setting, encouraging weaning or training the tantrum-ing toddler to regulate feelings and behaviour.

This conventional mode of paternal interaction buttresses the father's identity as a role-model of *collected composure in a risky situation*. Faced with the baby's hungry cravings, projectile vomiting or explosive poo, the father feels compelled to withdraw to defend against any threat of reactivated uncivilised weakness in himself. The early weeks of parenthood are dominated by his concern about coping with sleep deprivation, not only due to having to function efficiently at work, but anxiety of becoming more susceptible to facets of his own neediness or rage if exposed to the baby's wildness and mess. He regards the neonate as capable of loud, intentional, unappeasable and even spiteful demands and is concerned that these will encroach on his peace of mind. He firmly believes that regulation of the infant's sleep, crying and feeding patterns will constitute good training in learning boundaries. Another underlying unconscious threat, is due to anxiety about *scarcity of resources*. Underpinning this is *fear of the baby's insatiability* – a voracious capacity to fill every crevice of their space and deplete the family's financial or emotional assets, through excessive need or greed. So a predictable regime offers a framework to preserve the smooth running of the household and also provides reassuring anchorage during the confusing early weeks and months. Conversely, when the routine is breached it allows the infant's demands to encroach on spousal leisure time. A jealous Renouncer may exert scoffing superiority over the baby to counter retriggered feelings of being disregarded. Coping mechanisms tend towards the obsessional, and perinatal disturbance is likely to take a persecutory rather than depressive form.

Reciprocators

The Reciprocator father believes in a dynamic reciprocal adjustment rather than adapting to the infant (like the Participator father) or expecting the infant to adapt to the household (like the Renouncer). This means sizing up immediate happenings as they occur rather than following the predictable routine and task-oriented approach preferred by Renouncers, or habitual indulgence of the baby's needs as advocated by Participators.

Ultimately he takes a holistic view, alternating between self and others so as to meet his own needs while nurturing yet having to recognise needs different from his own. This self-other alternation differs from the Participator's selfless devotion in providing a perfect experience of infancy, or the Renouncer's focused determination to preserve his own efficiency in the adult world, unaffected by fatherhood. Reciprocator's anxieties relate to failing to respond to the complex needs of *all* family members which involves taking initiative and ongoing responsibility in shared care.

Prevalence of this category has increased in population surveys over the years. Initially in the early 1980s it appeared to be a mixture of the other two orientations. But in-depth interviews revealed this to be a separate approach with a philosophy of its own, rooted in *compassion* rather than identification – neither emulating a strong father figure like the Renouncer (with dis-identificatory detachment from nurturing mother and needy baby). Nor based on the Participator's identification with an idealised mother and/or infant.

A Reciprocator regards the baby as vulnerable yet robust, sentient from the start but prone to fluctuating 'states' of mind, with a rudimentary distinction between self and other. This differs from the Participator's belief that the fragile baby feels embedded in an undifferentiated symbiotic system, or the Renouncer's conviction that separate from birth, the powerful demanding baby is too self-centred to discriminate between carers.

In their anxiety to understand, Reciprocators must employ both ongoing *imagination* and a tolerance for *imperfection*. This is aided by accessibility of a medley of emotions. An 'open' father resonates to a spectrum of age-related feelings and admixture of (unproblematically assimilated) 'feminine' and 'masculine' qualities. If during pregnancy he was receptive to differences in the couple's male/female experience, sympathising with the discomforts of his pregnant woman while appreciating her willingness to carry their jointly conceived child, postnatally he remains aware of carer/baby emotional similarities while cognisant of their *experiential asymmetry*. So, at times his own states of mind vacillate between Participator-like experience of *'we-ness'* and Renouncer-like more distanced *'third-person'* view in observing the baby's actions. We may assume that this flexible ability to switch perspectives enhances empathy, allowing the Reciprocator to reflect on his own behaviour, to take note of mistakes and gauge the emotional effect he is having on his loved ones, and they on him.

In sum, this stance is a complex and difficult one, typified by willingness to improvise. This requires a mature capacity to tolerate uncertainty. Curious to see how the child will evolve he is not driven to influence development. Recognising the baby's sameness yet separateness, the Reciprocator father must both appreciate the newborn's sensitivity to hardships, and maintain trust in the vitality of growth. Above all, a Reciprocator father's awareness of *ambivalence* – both his own mixed feelings and those of other family members – allows their expression without having to split off, or project them.

Couple permutations

Most members of these three orientations make excellent fathers, who respond with appropriate warmth and care, when 'neither seduced nor frightened by the infant's needs and wishes' (as British psychoanalyst Ralph Layland wrote in 1981 about the capacity to be a loving father). As with mothers, problematic manifestations are found to reside in the extremes of either pole, or in the 'conflicted' mix of the two.

Needless to say, paternal orientations have their maternal corollaries – Facilitator, Regulator and Reciprocator mothers. In two parent families, the emotional climate of each joint household will largely depend on the specific combination of parental orientations and their couple dynamics.[5]

A Facilitator mother regards mothering as her exclusive domain. Adapting to the baby she feels uniquely primed by communion during pregnancy and breastfeeding to intuit the baby's symbiotic needs. Conversely, a Regulator mother expects the baby to adapt to the household. Since she regards mothering as a learned skill and the newborn as undiscriminating, she chooses to share care and implements a routine to provide continuity across co-carers. For the Regulator mother the primary entity remains the adult couple rather than the Facilitator's mother-baby unit.

Reciprocators, both male and female, try to hold in mind the needs of various members of the threesome or wider family, which necessitates negotiating each requirement as it arises, rather than imposing expert knowledge on the baby or always following his/her lead.

Different permutations of combined orientations manifest in a variety of parenting patterns, which seem to apply to same-sex couples too:

- A Participator father whose Regulator partner prefers to share care may be allocated the major share of nurturing, an arrangement that suits them both. But babies are expensive to maintain. His wish to be a full-time carer may be granted if her earnings can support the family, or if a Scandinavian-type fully-paid extended paternity leave is available. In some dual-income families both may work part-time, and/or from home. However, in such a coupling, the mother may resent the father's preoccupation with the infant if she feels it encroaches on their adult twosome, and while he disapproves of the routine she advocates, she begrudges his 'indulgence' rather than setting limits.
- Conversely, a Participator father espoused to a Facilitator mother may vie competitively over primary caregiving, particularly if each craves sole responsibility. Some couples achieve an amicable division of care *('I change nappies; she baths the baby and we share the feeds').* But if breast-feeding is the exclusive form of nourishment, he may feel cheated and compelled to sabotage the envied intimacy. In this couple, for the duration of the infancy their prime bond is to the baby, and in many cases their sexual relationship is put on hold for a year or more by the baby in their bed.
- In a household composed of a Renouncer father and Facilitator mother they agree that as the traditional breadwinner he is not expected to participate in

baby-care, which they both acknowledge as her own exclusive domain. However, they may clash if he is unable to provide the supportive emotional and practical backing she requires to achieve the ideal kind of facilitation she aspires to particularly if there are other young children in the family who need care, or if he finds her breastfeeding distasteful, or fears losing out on her affection, now centred on the new baby.

- If by contrast, a traditional Renouncer father is espoused to a Regulator and expects her to be a stay-at-home mother while she prefers to be out there working in the adult world, she may develop persecutory feelings of paranoia or resentment. Similarly, a Renouncer/Regulator couple who lack practical support and cannot afford to pay, face unwelcome compromises and experience persecutory distress at enforced childcare. Thus, in each household, the precipitants of postnatal disturbance vary according to orientation, triggered by obstacles to meeting their own ideal expectations of parenting.
- At the extremes, Participator fathers and Facilitator mothers may be so over-identified that the baby has difficulty individuating. Extreme Renouncer fathers and Regulator mothers may be so aloof (to avoid contagious resonance) that they detach from/dismiss their responsive feelings.
- Finally, a Reciprocator with any partner is likely to accept differences in their baby-care styles, and tolerates the healthy ambivalence of parenting. As noted, rather than treating the sexual couple or carer-infant as a primary unit, spontaneity necessitates maintaining a broader overview beyond the dyad and the Reciprocator focuses on creative ways of working as a family, regarded as an interlocking system of relations. As this moniker suggests through reciprocal engagement while trying to help the baby to make sense of the world, the Reciprocator comes to self-discovery.

Discussion: beliefs and biases

In my experience, it is useful for research studies to delineate different subgroups as these tend to cancel each other out in more generalised findings. For instance, compared with non-fathers, dads are said to report higher levels of happiness, positive emotion and meaning in life (Nelson, Kushlev, English, Dunn, & Lyubomirsky, 2013). And recent studies stress that fathers are just as likely as mothers to see parenting as extremely important to their identity. Micro-analyses of filmed observations show that fathers can be as perceptive, caring and competent as mothers in raising a child.

Moreover, paternal physiological responses resemble those of caregiving mothers – heart rate and blood pressure rise with the baby's cry or smiles.[6] However, as this chapter notes all along, fathers are not all alike and such generalisations overlook gradations and do not distinguish between different types of responses. Delineating different orientations my own studies (tautologically) show less engrossment or desire for emotional engagement in men of a Renouncer orientation, who define their role as fostering autonomy and self-control in the child. Stressing the positive ignores the fact that some parents come to regret having had children. Likewise, studies that pose a dichotomy ignore the spectrum. For instance, insisting that parental play differs by sex. Thus rough-and-tumble play is ascribed to (American) fathers. This 'disruptively attuned' exciting approach is seen to develop curiosity, problem solving skills and assertiveness by challenging the child's expectations (Herzog, 1998). However, when qualitative research links sensitivity to cues and responsive attunement not to gender but to the carer's *familiarity* through hours of contact with the child, in primary carer fathers the nature of play is found to be soothing, more like that of stay-at-home mothers (Field, 1978; Pruett & Litzenberger, 1992).

Observations show that mothers who return from work outside the home, are also likely to greet the child with enthusiastic, stimulating play. Delineating specific *subgroups of fathers* helps compare and contrast, refining understanding and dispelling some untested preconceptions. For instance, the sweeping assumption that fathers respond more flirtatiously to little girls was made in heterosexual families. Research matching homosexual and heterosexual families not only did not encounter the anticipated gender problems, but found more positive parenting and parental well-being in gay father families. Further research *within* same-sex parent families, also pinpointed other protective factors (see Golombok, 2017). In psychoanalysis, too, binary theoretical generalisations obscured the fine details in Psychoanalysis too. Freud's emphasis on 'psychic bisexuality' was lost, and the father's importance overturned with Object Relations theorists' stress on maternal primacy, which also obfuscated the significance of the [pre-Oedipal] father's 'earliest role' (as Abelin noted in 1975). I argue that these psychoanalytic lacunae are not surprising, given a tendency to essentialise baby-care as female by unconsciously conflating womb with postnatal maternal 'containment'.

In my view, this metaphor has not only fed unrealistic expectations of seamless unambivalent mothering, but severely limited the conception of 'paternal function'. Blind spots have consequences. As long as the mother is viewed as an on-tap unconditionally delivering placenta – the role of the father must be confined to 'cord-cutting' to rescue the child from maternal 'engulfment'.[7]

Conversely, today, new research questions are being engendered by the evolving spectrum of non-cohabiting, same-sex and co-parenting fathers. Studies must try to tease out what it is that really matters in parenting: whether it is vitally important to have *two* parents, and if so, is the male/female duo essential? Or is it the *quality* of co-parenting that is crucial rather than the sex, orientation or type of paternal relation as Golombok found. What is it that defines a successful parental combination? Can dismissed (or 'dissed') fathers be reintegrated, both in theory and the home (see Gorell Barnes, 2017)? Might a relative, nanny or other type of 'allo-carer' serve as the second responsible adult, not necessarily formulated as an additional 'father' or 'mother'? Is there an ideal way of fathering or co-pairing of orientations? Many unanswered questions remain. My own contribution has been to look to the complex origins of a subjective desire to be a parent and how a spectrum of such underpinnings tend to play out over time in practice.

Demographic changes

If today financial independence enables some women to choose to mother alone (conceiving by ART or discharging the biological father from the fold), an analogous contemporary innovation is that of *single fatherhood by choice.* But paternal childrearing in itself is not a new phenomenon. Historically it was remarkably prevalent – in pre-industrial Britain (between 1599 and 1811) almost *a* quarter of all children lived in families with a lone father![8] In fact, homes only became matri-centric during the 19th century while Britain was the manufacturing centre of Europe. Occupying territory on four different continents, the vast trading and commercial empire required its men to work abroad or in centralised factories and mass workplaces a long commute from home. In addition to market forces, the extremely divergent emotional experience of fathers and mothers during both World Wars further contributed to men's secondary role in childcare, both while away and on their return.

My contention is that in each era, *prescribed parental roles* follow a politically motivated form of theorising about the needs of babies, how these are best met and by whom. In historical periods when less personal choice prevails, governmental dictates designate specialist 'gurus' to coach parents to raise the future citizens needed by the state. These advocate either strict disciplinary regulatory measures (e.g. Truby King) or permissive facilitatory ideologies of childcare (Spock, Winnicott, Bowlby), which suit the particular demographic and material circumstances of each era.

But a massive change occurred when the sixties' counter-culture began to challenge binary stereotypes and demand that birth-chambers opened their doors to fathers. I ascribe today's rising incidence of greater paternal involvement to many factors, not least the fact that two or three generations of western children have already benefitted from more hands-on caregiving by their fathers.

In tandem with proliferating maternal choices, mass media now poses fatherhood as a more prominent feature of men's identity. But as noted, this varies in practice across the range of paternal orientations. Couple dynamics enter into the picture and if many fathers seem more enthusiastically engaged, for some this now also involves taking more initiative with a longer unsupervised period of parenting activity before they are monitored (usually by the mother). Borrowing a term used by Elliott Jaques for the work-place, we may call this new responsibility a paternal 'time-span of discretion'.[9]

Western cultural imagery around masculinity continues to change apace. Previous social norms emphasised *male dominance* – heroic risk-taking; sexual promiscuity; alpha-male rivalry and power over women. However, macho constraint on expression of intimate feelings has proven toxic, associated with high rates of cardiovascular disease, substance abuse, poor social functioning, bullying and mental ill-health in competitive men who strive to conform to the high-powered A-prototype. The broadening categorisation of gender characteristics which tenderised fatherhood were also associated with liberalised attitudes towards homosexuality.[10] Systemic sexism and abuse by rank is being outed by current anti-harassment movements (e.g. '#TimesUp' and '#Me Too'). And even princes, celebrities, firefighters and policemen now publicly admit to feeling traumatised, sharing painful experiences that erode the persistent myth of male impermeability to shock, sadness and depression.

So, against a backdrop of technological advances alterations in fatherhood can be ascribed to multifaceted demographic modifications over the past century. Urbanisation and a vastly accelerated pace of life due to widespread economic migration and enforced social mobility has weakened extended family ties. Greater population density and diversity in sprawling mega-cities is characterised by pluricultural variation with rapidly changing sexual and social mores. Crucially for fatherhood, city-dwelling usually entails alienation and lowered social cohesiveness (as predicted by Durkheim), and intense reliance on fewer, yet more complex, intimate relationships. But I suggest that urban anonymity also fosters non-conformity and greater freedom to apply one's personal preferences, with far-reaching implications for parenting.

In a super-sized hyper-disparate city people's experience varies tremendously even within a single district. In London (considered to be the most diverse mega-city in the world with over 300 spoken languages), paternal orientation is affected by differences of temperament, sexuality, class, race, ethnicity, education and income. Some fathers are gregarious with large interconnected social networks, while other fathers seek a less outgoing, more insular way of life, perhaps embedded in a close, or even closed, community. Not surprisingly, the spectrum of emotional engagement in fatherhood varies, too, spanning deep engrossment to disavowal, or even active flight. Furthermore, in pluralist societies, besides inter-generational fractures, a potential clash exists between dominant social expectancies and each father's own normative subculture. Further discrepancies arise between mass- or social media depictions of fatherhood, and what takes place in the privacy of the home. Not surprisingly then, paternal engagement not only varies cross-culturally, but even in the same location multiple patterns of parenting exist among fathers, and also within each father over time. Variations in empathy occur even within the self-same paternal figure due to shifting attention or temporary distraction: *'Fucking morons!'* a father barks into his smartphone, unmindful how his visibly shocked infant flinches at the rough whip of his voice . . .[11]

Moreover, today some 20–25% of European women now choose to forgo motherhood altogether, content to apply their generative agency in occupational fields other than reproduction. As a result, in some countries the birth rate has fallen below the critical replacement rate of 2.2 (to 1.9 in the UK and 1.34 in

Italy!) Other women who postpone childbearing while engaging in education and/or a satisfying career may encounter age-reduced fertility. Similarly, virility declines in older men. But life style changes have generated an unprecedented threat – in Australia, North America and Europe sperm count has dropped even in younger men by more than 50% in less than 40 years! A meta-study of 43,000 men ascribes sperm decline to environmental toxicants, excessive alcohol, obesity, drug intake and rising comorbidities in regions of accelerated industry. Researchers now predict that if this trend continues, by 2050 the sperm count of Western men will be zero (Levine et al., 2017). *Begetting would be confined to sperm banks!*

In conclusion

We live in unusual times when fathers are burgeoning while fathering is threatened and, no longer prescribed, paternal practice is open to personal interpretations. Viewing the vicissitudes of fatherhood from a variety of interleaving theoretical perspectives – historical, socio-cultural, psycho-sexual, psychoanalytic and philosophical – this chapter has charted the effect of changing male/female stereotypes and prototypes of masculinity. I claim that in the past, specific child-care ideologies fluctuated to meet politico-economic necessities, drawing in each era on commensurate myths, studies and stereotypes to enforce compliance. Thus encouraging conformity with strict gender roles served a political socio-economic function in its time, reinforcing advantageous power hierarchies. In retrospect we see how regulatory baby-regimentation was apposite for instituting a female workforce during the wars and the Great Depression; and that the sea-change to facilitatory maternal devotion in the home suited the post war years of returning soldiers.

To my mind, we may ascribe some of today's new wave of more engaged fathers across the spectrum to open disillusionment with authority figures who spawned a world of increasing uncertainties and feared dangers for their children. Patriarchal omnipotence has been further punctured in the wake of 9/11, and exposure of man-made global disasters accelerate distrust with complacent, unreliable, power-seeking or fraudulent governance. The art of being a father now means striving to impart security.

In these hazardous times some parents express an urgent need for expert guidance and child-care gurus proliferate with contradictory advice. Others feel that all any loving parent can hope to do to counteract unreliable leaders and environmental risks is to take responsibility for improving their child's future – each according to their own beliefs, needs and chosen orientation.

Notes

1 According to the Families and Work Institute in New York City dads now provide three-quarters of the types of childcare that mothers do (up from one-half thirty

years ago). US statistics indicate more than two million primary-care fathers (whether by choice, or of necessity due to rising male unemployment). In the UK, dissatisfied with their 'work/home balance' many same-sex and heterosexual fathers are inventing novel ways to spend more time with the child. 94% of fathers take some time off work when their child is born, and a third of them supplement the statutory two weeks with their holiday entitlement to spend more time with their family. However, three years after its introduction, less than 2% of UK fathers take up *shared* parental leave. This compares with 90% of fathers in Sweden, where 80–100% of their earnings are replaced while they are on leave. Nonetheless, many western men do seem keen to be more engaged, and if the last few decades saw a rise in single mothers (choosing to raise a child born of unexpected conception or actively planning donor insemination), some men too now decide to become solo fathers through adoption or surrogate gestation.

2 Today's young people have expanded gender categories. These range from non-conflicted fluidity across previously dichotomised 'masculine/feminine' characteristics, to transgender identification with the other sex (and possibly, transsexual physical 'transitioning').

Nonconformist categories such as 'bi-gender' self-identify as male and female at different times; 'androgynes' who see themselves as a separate, third gender blending both male and female characteristics (akin to the 'hijira' in India and Pakistan) or 'agender/neutrois' who identify with no gender. In a climate of greater social tolerance of early gender experimentation, even the Church of England recently encouraged its teachers to accept cross-dressing in their primary schools. And the Tavistock Gender Identity Clinic now has referrals of children as young as four wanting to change sex.

3 Social, philosophical and legal issues regarding moral constraints on the means of procreation and parental roles, rights and responsibilities are beyond the scope of this chapter. Suffice to say here that biology can no longer serve as the sole determinant of paternity as demonstrated by state intervention when guardians exceed limits or fail to meet their obligations. Ethically, legislation must also limit the number of families served by any single sperm donor (internet searches in the USA discover 50+ half-siblings).

4 State provisions reveal a society's main concerns which impact on family function. Shared care is more likely from the start when the importance of *all* members of the family is acknowledged. For instance, in Denmark for decades hospitals have provided rooming-in facilities (with a double bed) for the father and other children to stay over after the birth. In general, Denmark and the other Scandinavian countries, Iceland, Finland, Norway, Sweden top the 2014 world's gender equality index, with generous parental leave to care for sick children and reduced job-travel demands and family-friendly work hours. The civilised 4pm end of the working day enables fathers to participate in fun and games as well as housework, homework and bedtime rituals. Swedish fathers, who receive the most lavish paternity leave (480 days shared by the couple) spend more than ten times (!) per week with their infants as American or UK fathers, and as much time as mothers in dual-earning families.

5 Longitudinal treatment with 'dysfunctional families' shows that improving the mother and father's relationship is the best predictor of well-adjusted children. Group couple discussions (Cowan, 1996), new parent diaries (Burgess, 1997), and study observations (Lewis, 1986) reveal how *partner dynamics* tacitly affect parenting patterns, suggesting that fathers often hold back while mothers guard their domain by undermining paternal self-confidence. In fact, studies pinpoints two important factors associated with fatherhood: *supportive co-parenting and couple*

intimacy. Research finds that fathers who have a good relationship with the baby's mother are more likely to be responsive, confident and affectionate towards the child. A higher level of spousal intimacy is correlated with a more secure father-infant attachment relationship, while deteriorating intimacy is correlated with negative father-child interaction. (Belsky, Youngblade, Rovine, & Volling, 1991). Not surprisingly, paternal and maternal disturbance are also strongly correlated within the family dynamic system in which the emotional experience of each member affects all others in various ways. Paternal perinatal disturbance is high (invariably over-diagnosed as postnatal 'depression' rather than distinguishing 'persecutory' elements as I have advocated here). It rises to a quarter of new fathers between three and six months postpartum, a prevalence approaching that of maternal disturbance (Paulson & Bazemore, 2010). Depressive symptoms in new fathers are significantly associated with perinatal distress of the partner and found to predict poor child emotional and psychological development as well as child psychopathology and behavioural problems, independently of maternal depression (Ramchandani et al., 2011). My research has specified varying precipitants of perinatal emotional disturbance that differ with orientation, and reflect a subjective response to the discrepancy between each father's own ideals and thwarted expectations. (Raphael-Leff, 1985).

6 While fathers do not undergo the endocrine changes of gestation and lactation that 'prime' maternality in women, infant stimulated hormonal changes are seen to occur in 'hands on' fathers, who have higher levels of oestrogen (the female 'sex hormone') and oxytocin than other men, and non-engaged fathers. These hormonal changes occur in *response* to cuddling or hearing a baby cry, rather than instigating paternal behaviour. Cohabiting fathers show reductions in testosterone during the first three weeks after the birth when the hormone drops by a third, seemingly an adaptive response leading to decreased 'fight or flight' behaviours facilitating greater focus on the baby due to reduced sex-drive, inhibiting competitiveness and aggression (Brizendine, 2010; Rilling, 2013).

7 For decades conservative caution prevailed, resulting in sparse psychoanalytic literature on fathers. Even a panel on 'the role of the father in the preoedipal years' referred uneasily to 'the recent blurring of maternal and paternal roles and increased participation by fathers in the nurturing of their children' (Kramer & Prall, 1978). Dogmatically, it reiterated the essential paternal provision of 'a shield' to the child, especially the son, against the mother's wish to prolong 'symbiosis'. But in tandem with feminism, exploration of the effects of father absence resulted in a burgeoning of awareness of paternal input (Glasser, 1985; Lamb, 1975; Ross, 1979) and 'hunger' for a real relationship and its loving manifestation (Herzog, 1982; Layland, 1981). In time, psychoanalytic studies began noting dynamics between the 'internal', symbolic and *real* external father; and from a Jungian perspective 'contrasexual' anima/animus projections. Yet even today the pre-Oedipal father is often still posited as a mere 'paternal integer' in the maternal mind. When orthodoxy prevails despite 21st-century thought-provoking new patterns of father-care, 19th-century psychoanalytic gender stereotypy persists. The very concept of triangulation, ever-attributed to that classical 'paternal function' of separating 'merged' mother and infant, disregarded both the scope of women for such 'thirdness', and the existence of enmeshed father-baby dyads. Even a contemporary psychoanalytic 're-evaluation' of the importance of fathers (Etchegoyen, 2002) treats with caution the 'extreme view' that maternal/paternal functions are not necessarily sex-related (Samuels, 1996). In addition, psychoanalytic concentration on *dyadic* mother-baby pairs had other theoretical repercussions – occluding ordinary *triadic* attachment. In due course attachment researchers rescinded Bowlby's original dictum of a

monotropic bond, noting that infants actually have the capacity for *multiple* primary attachments rather than exclusively to the mother. But recognition of the neonate's early capacity to relate *simultaneously* to two or more carers was severely delayed, and only conceded at the turn of this century due to undeniable cumulative observational and scientific evidence (Fivaz-Depeursinge & Corboz-Warnery 1999; Klitzing, Simoni, & Bürgin, 1999).

8 While today some fathers are depicted as 'new men' by contrast to remote, authoritarian fathers of the past, recent research has revealed a discrepancy between that public face of patriarchal fatherhood advocated by Church and 'advice literature', and private emotional experience. Autobiographies and personal journals of fathers over the past few hundred years reveal that in pre-industrialised societies where the home was the workplace, with little separation between adult and child space, fathers often engaged in daily 'cradle-side' childcare as well as domestic work (Laslett, 1983). Furthermore, high maternal morbidity in childbirth left many babies motherless, and widowers often remained single rather than remarry. They tended not to engage another female to take care of the baby, especially if there were unmarried daughters in the family. In addition, divorcing men were automatically given custody of the children and due to low life expectancy, grandparents were usually no longer alive to offer assistance, so fathers often had to involve themselves directly in childcare. Finally, their letters and diaries often expressed tender feelings for live offspring (e.g. James Boswell and Thomas More) and profound grief for those who died (e.g. Ben Jonson, cited by Burgess, 1997).

9 I want to emphasise the marked difference between a father's 'involvement' in day to day tasks of feeding, bathing, reading, soothing, nappy changing etc. vs. *initiating* these or taking on full responsibility for the ongoing welfare of the child. Among European fathers today, equality indicators show that the *duration* of father-care is still much lower than that of mothers. British men spend an average of 24 minutes caring for children for every hour done by women, the lowest of 15 countries for which there was data for this indicator. In Portugal, where the ratio is highest, men do 60% more childcare: but still only 39 minutes for every hour done by women. Increasingly in many low income countries, various organisations worldwide now run community-based fatherhood groups to raise paternal involvement. For instance, the MenCare Global Fatherhood campaign has reached 250,000 men in over 25 countries on five continents since its establishment in 2011, providing opportunities for fathers to discuss personal experience, learn practical caregiving and communication skills, and positive discipline methods (eschewing corporal punishment).

This is very salient across the African continent, where many traditions define fathers almost exclusively as material providers (and punitive authoritarians), and unemployed or low earning fathers tend to be excluded (or opt out) from seeing their kids.

10 Even macho Australia has just legitimised same-sex marriage although as I write 33 African countries operate laws that criminalise 'queerness', an anti-gay stance shared in parts of the Middle East and Asia still characterised by macho ideology or dogmatic religious morality.

11 My model reflects personal predilections which are more consciously expressed in contemporary multicultural urbanised societies where greater choice prevails. Settled rural populations in the same country may follow local religious or tradition conventions which over-ride personal choice. Conflict between generations often rests on beliefs about gender roles and the needs of babies. Where tribal customs prevail as in parts of modern day South Africa, despite urban 'modernisation', the first child may

still have to be given to the paternal grandmother. Similarly, first generation seemingly acculturated immigrants in large European cities tend in their private domain to adhere to ways of their culture of origin (e.g., seclusion rules, special nutrition and rules about timing of post-parturition resumption of sex), that may clash with local prescriptions or are eroded in the next generation. Finally, in some conformist cultures normative practice leans sequentially towards toward one or other pole of the model (e.g. in Japan early facilitator 'skinship' is replaced at age two by strict maternal regulation).

Chapter 7

Working with the triad

Tessa Baradon

Daniel Stern made the following observation on 'the triad' in his progress report on the clinical relevance of infancy (2008):

> I must say that (until I met the Lausanne group) I considered a triad to be nothing more than *three dyads at play at the same time*. It took me a long time to realize that there is another entity called 'the triad'. I think that my difficulty was not particular to me. Many of us who work with the dyad do not appreciate the *systemic reality of triads*, such as mother-father-baby or mother-baby-therapist.

The principle that the therapeutic work encompasses all the participants in the encounter requires that, at different times in the session and across the course of meetings, the therapy moves between individual, dyadic, triadic and systemic foci. The individual work addresses the internal worlds of baby, mother and father respectively. These are also expressed in the attributes and conflicts they bring to the arena of interactions. Attention to the 'three dyads at play (or at work) at the same time' looks at the bi-directional quality of interactions and influences in the mother-infant, father-infant, and mother-father. In other words, how each dyad choreographs their particular dance. Their 'systemic' reality applies to their coming together as a family. It includes the interactions between all three as well as dyadic interactions with a third in mind. Thus, the presence of the triad offers a possibility of addressing environmental provision for each member in relation to the other, and as a unit. This notion of environmental provision extends Winnicott's idea of maternal environmental provision for the baby – all aspects the infant's physical and psychological care and his/her experience of this (Winnicott, 1960, p. 592). Indeed, in the triadic setting the primary relationships of the baby with his mother, his father and their coupledom, and what infant needs from each parent in the context of his/her relationship with the other, are more explicit and available for reflection and reframing (clinical illustrations of this are discussed in Chapters 4 and 11). Thought can also be given to the patterns of nurturance between the adults and in their support for each other's relationship with their baby. These are critical to the sense of safety and creativity of the family.

However, the presence of mother and father together in a therapeutic session with their baby is also challenging. Not only is it a psychological stretch for the therapist to attend to three bodies, minds, ghosts etc., which present a contemporaneous flow of narratives and needs. Indeed, even experienced therapists can feel overloaded by the totality of material and the dynamics of the family system in a session. There are also potential challenges specifically associated with the father's physical presence. I will address in this chapter: engaging with a triad, the 'libidinal group' and the positioning of the therapist within this group, and challenges in processing sexuality and couple issues in the parent-infant psychotherapy therapeutic encounter.

Establishing an agreed frame for engaging with the triad

Introduction to the frame of parent-infant psychotherapy is itself different from setting the frame in other analytic modalities inasmuch as it is a mixed infant and adult led space, involving emotional, embodied reverberations with infantile states (for a description of the frame and steps to engagement, see Baradon, 2016; Biseo, 2016). Some fathers may immediately be interested and even feel relief and gratitude at the recognition of their struggles as father, or with their partner's mothering, or with their baby's personality and behaviours. An example of this was a phone call from a first-time father to the Anna Freud Centre, explaining that his wife and baby were due to be discharged from a psychiatric mother and baby inpatient unit, and they needed 'help to become a family'. Another example was a man who asked his partner 'check the therapist out' and then came to the following session and attended regularly thereafter. Other fathers, however, may exclude themselves from therapy for a longer period, or attend intermittently. I have found that such irregular arrangements can work for the family if the frame is agreed by both parents and the entrances and departures are thought about. In time it may take on the rhythm and meaning of the father's ordinary coming and going such as, for example, if he is the working parent leaving and returning to the home over the course of the day.

There are different ways for fathers to position themselves in relation to the therapy, thus impacting the ways in which they participate in the process. Some arrangements stay more with a focus on mother and baby as the normative clients and others look to be more genuinely inclusive of father's own needs and aspirations. In each case, the father himself may have his own preference depending on his needs, defences and his accommodation to the overt and implicit wishes of his partner. Maintaining the engagement of both parents in parent-infant psychotherapy requires genuinely agreeing the rationale and frame for *shared* work, whichever forms it takes. I will give examples of each, although a 'true form' of each approach is rarely adhered to (and appropriately so), and the frame may change over time.

Working with mother and baby 'in the presence of' the father

It remains the case that in many instances the concern of professionals is the perinatal mental health of the mother and she is the identified patient. It is often hoped that the father can function as the emotional prop for mother, and buffer for the baby. The parents may indeed present in the first session with an expectation that father has come to support his partner, and father's participation may have been secured on this basis. While this may work over time for some families, in my experience it is often the case that the father drifts away from the therapy as soon as there are signs of improvement in his partner. The following is a case which illustrates this.

A midwife was alerted to high levels of depression in a mother soon after giving birth and referred the mother for parent-infant psychotherapy. The therapist invited the mother to bring the father, and he did attend. He was very worried about his wife and reassuring towards her. In the session he was the one who responded tenderly to the baby. It was early days, mother was deeply unwell, and the therapist was very concerned for her, and for the tiny, dependent baby. She reinforced the measures the family had taken whereby father looked after the two vulnerable members. Father agreed to continue to attend sessions in this role but soon the burdens of work and caretaking took precedence. Initially he dropped mother and baby at the centre and then went on to do the chores, then mother was well enough to come without his help. The therapist worked with mother and baby and after six months or so, mother's depression had lifted, and the case was closed.

In supervision, when discussing the work, the therapist spoke about mother's problematic past, her issues of identity, the meaning of the pregnancy and baby for her, the observed relationship with the baby in the room. She described her work with the 'baby as a subject' (Thomson-Salo & Paul, 2007) and the baby's emergent personality and development. But when asked about father, she had little to say. She did not know how he felt about becoming a father, his partner's collapse and the unexpected emotional adaptations he had to make.

This case illustrates further potential dynamics when Mother is the identified patient and father positioned as 'the coping parent'. Particularly in situations of crisis, the father 'as subject' is easily overlooked. In this way he may become stuck in an idealised position as the locus of health for the family, as much as the mother is trapped in her 'failure' as mother and as partner. Worried (and often overloaded) professionals may collude with the notion of an all-capable father, such that even limited thought about his current state is occluded and an opportunity for therapeutic support for him is missed. Often, over time, his participation becomes tokenistic or falters. Furthermore, the split representations of strong and frail parent risk becoming ossified at the expense of growth of the couple as parents. However, if space can be made for the father's experience, and is accepted by him, more collaborative outcomes can be achieved.

Working with a series of dyads

Working with dyadic parent-infant issues may be the aim of the work, or may be a phase of therapy that then extends to triadic aspects. When both parents are burdened with psychological issues, attending to the individual parental needs and their relationship with the baby may be what is manageable. The following case illustrates therapeutic work with a father-baby dyad.

Father was illegally in the country, destitute and homeless. Yet he continued to be present in his daughter's daily life. Not surprisingly, given both his early history of abuse and his lack of agency regarding his current life circumstances, he was also extremely passive in his parenting endeavour. An early aim of the therapy was to help father to express his emotional claim of his infant more actively.

In the second session Lila, age eight months, cried intermittently. Initially her mother comforted her; when she cried again the therapist asked her father to respond. The father picked up a toy train and rattled it to draw Lila's attention. She looked at him and the train. He started driving it slowly towards her, and the therapist picked up the thread verbally: 'Daddy is driving the train, it is coming clo-s-e-r' (voice rises as Lila shimmers), Lila is interested – she is watching, 'O she's not sure – is the train going too fast, she is asking daddy what will happen next . . .'. Her father started monitoring Lila's responses and moving the train accordingly – pausing when she seemed uncertain and proceeding when she was ready. Mother watched with a faint smile. A few minutes later Lila was ensconced on her father's lap, the train no longer needed to mediate their linking. The therapist reflected her thoughts about the father's choice of the toy train as symbolic of his arrival in the UK with no one to help him to make safe connections with this new country, and his wish to provide a safe emotional environment for his daughter. This elicited a profound response in father to which mother listened with compassion.

Key in the above example are the interventions to support the father's and the baby's agency in reaching out to each other. It reframed each as an interesting and effective partner to the other. In tandem, more general principles of sensitivity – observing the baby's/other's cues, interpreting them meaningfully and responding contingently – were being established as a familial frame for relating. When the joining up of father and daughter had taken place, the therapist moved to interpret some of the unconsoled cries in the father that were played out in his interactions with his child. This interpretation was meaningful also to Lila's mother, and emotionally linked the parents.

Working with the triad

Cowan & Cowan (1987) propose that 'fathering is a family affair'. The role the father plays with his child emerges from a complex, circular interaction pattern in which each family domain affects and is affected by all of the others' (p. 165). The influences of the father on the mother-infant dyad, of the mother on the father-infant dyad, and the baby on the couple are multi-directional. They can work toward splitting and exclusion, as illustrated in the clinical chapters in this book, or towards 'a truly interactive triad in which positive marital communication and stimulating, positive and responsive mothering and fathering can occur' (Belsky & Volling 1987, p. 54).

The struggle to become a creative triad can be brought to the consulting room overtly or implicitly. This struggle seems most apparent in families where the birth of the baby has placed contradictory sets of stresses on the parents, individually and as a couple. On the one hand, there is the wish and the need to protect and nurture the vulnerable and dependent infant who is, henceforth, their responsibility. On the other hand, the infant's survival and healthy development seem to have required too much narcissistic compromise on the part of the parent/s. For some parents, and some couples, this has led to persecutory and rivalrous fantasies, and the couple relationship and/or that with the baby have become the playgrounds for these conflicts. The parents and baby may need the therapist to help them to discover their potential meeting point. Palacio Espasa & Knauer (2007) discusses shared unconscious elements, such as fantasies and projections that can form 'a common interpretative focus' (p. 68) to promote engagement.

For example, over the early months of therapy (family above) the therapist witnessed first mother, then father, become severely depressed. She spoke with each about their mood and underpinning experiences, past and present. In the following vignette she addressed triadic aspects.

Lila, aged 11 months, crawled over to the therapist at the beginning of the session and placed herself chest-to-chest, leaning into to her and breathing heavily. The therapist said softly to Lila that she was telling her therapist and her parents something important about how she was feeling very sad and lonely. Lila's parents initially dismissed her behaviour as 'clingy', but the therapist persisted with the idea that her behaviour had emotional meaning. The parents become curious and remembered other examples of Lila needing 'reassurance' from them. The therapist then made a link with their respective episodes of depression:

> I wonder whether when each of you is depressed you are physically present but you aren't with each other or with her in your minds. Is that a bit of a theme for all of you, and especially Lila who is so small: that you are present but also she can lose both of you to depression?

Both parents looked distressed but discussed this thoughtfully. Lila turned to face them as they spoke, looking from one to the other. She then moved away from the therapist – first to the mother's lap and then to the father's.

This vignette illustrates triadic work in which experiences of depression and withdrawal in each individual were thought about in terms of the family system, including the baby – who in this session had shed her clowning behaviour and was communicating her depression and withdrawal. It drew upon previous psychological exploration with mother and father as individuals, as well as their collaboration in co-parenting. The common interpretative focus was on the triad's defensive response to the 'bad world'. Research confirms that couple discussion of child related issues increases paternal involvement (Cowan & Cowan, 1987) and, for this family, such conversations took place only in the emotionally safe environment of the consulting room.

Triadic parent-infant psychotherapy can also include discussions about the couple relationship, with the therapist tasked to keep the baby in mind when, in the pull towards conflict, s/he is forgotten by the parents. The baby's presence in the room enables parents and therapist to receive immediate information from him/her about the impact of the parental relationship and the aspects with which the infant struggles. This may help them to recognise their baby's sentience to their relationship and promote awareness of his/her experience and its procedural encoding. Emanuel and Von Klitzing discuss couple work in this volume. Salomonsson (2018a) reinforces the baby's place in parent-infant psychotherapy

> Babies have a talent of attracting our attention and readiness to engage. In therapy, they exert this 'magnet' function by forcing the parents to approach a problem which, if unsolved, can jeopardize his future. To phrase it differently, he brings out more adult parts of his parents' personalities.
>
> (Salomonsson, 2018a, p. 117)

A libidinal group and the position of the therapist therein: a change in the nature and experience of the work

In dyadic mother-infant psychotherapy the therapist often occupies the role of the third, often carrying the 'paternal function' (IPA Debates, 2014). This can be summed up as a reflective mind that enables simultaneous containment of the mother-infant dyad and their separateness. This paradox can be delicately scaffolded by the therapist joining with the mother – as the two adults in the room and in the transference – to present a thinking couple in relation to the baby. This may be a 'parental couple' coming together around the baby. Alternately, it may be the 'motherhood constellation' in which the therapist is transferentially positioned as the nurturing (grand)mother who offers the mother and the baby an experience of being contained transgenerationally (Stern, 1995).

This in-side/out-side position can affect the experiences of intimacy in the therapeutic encounter for the mother and the therapist. In my view, it can be hard for both mother and therapist to surrender the transference intimacy of dyadic work and sometimes this can be an obstacle to including fathers in the therapy and working with the nuclear family triad. The libidinal group may also bring more conflictual hue to the transferences, such as sibling rivalries, the shifting sands of inclusive and exclusive sub-groupings, issues around favouritism and neglect and other negative forces within that attack the family as an attachment unit. The ability to tolerate such assaults is a critical part of this work.

The not-often-spoken-about: sexuality in the room

Having father, mother and the baby in the room together, particularly very soon after birth, potentially introduces sexuality in a very direct way. The baby is a concrete representation of intercourse and introduces the couple's real sexuality and fecundity into the consulting room. Moreover, the baby brings an immediacy of psychological-visceral experiences which permeate the fabric of the session: fluids, odours, excretions, mess, appetite and emotional vehemence – all evocative of (the recent) intercourse.

Frequently it is sexuality overshadowed by exhaustion that presents in the consulting room, a recalled aspect of the coupledom now cobwebbed by sleeplessness and anxiety. Sometimes sparks emerge in the course of routine care of the baby, who can himself/herself be a trigger to sensuous/sensual feelings in the adult, since nurturing an infant includes so much potentially erotic bodily contact – softness, rounded limbs, mouthing. An example was reported by a PIP therapist-in-training:

Mother was breast-feeding her baby boy. While suckling, the infant slowly handled her breast. He seemed suffused with pleasurable corporeal experience. The trainee reported entering a kind of reverie, enveloped in the palpable sensuality of the infant's feed. She imagined the warm mild liquid flowing into his mouth, soothing his gums, reaching his stomach, expanding into a feeling of security and wellbeing. Her immersed state of identification was suddenly disrupted when the father, who was watching his wife and infant, exclaimed 'jokingly': 'Hey, those [breasts] are mine!'. With the father's interjection the trainee suddenly felt extremely uncomfortable, as though she was treading a fine line between self-exposure through identification, professional interest as an observer, and voyeurism – where exposure to the sexual lives of others carries connotations of 'peeping' and transgression.

This vignette brings alive the intense embodied emotional responses in all participants. Perhaps the baby's suckling acted as a mnemonic to earliest visceral memories of passion, eroticism and satiation in each of the adults. The father's presence interpolated the 'real' into the more common analytic currency of fantasy. His erotic interjection was experienced by the trainee as breaking the idyllic/idealised boundary between mother and infant and the outside world, by introducing the union of the couple. Her feelings of sudden exclusion and of transgression reflect meeting the reality of the 'outsider within' dilemma discussed above.

Sexuality can evolve as the focal point in the therapy. It may underpin the couple's difficulties in their transition into parenthood, such as when a mother's engrossment with her baby is perceived by father as channelling her sexual interest away from him. In other cases, it may be 'used' as a defence against the therapeutic work. The example below illustrates this.

The mother was the referred patient with personality disorder. The father accompanied his wife and four week baby girl to the session. While the mother spoke in whispers about her experience of the baby as a parasite, Father used his booming voice to pronounce on his wife's 'mental illness'. The therapist was shocked by the emaciated appearance of the mother and her sense of being hollowed out by her tiny baby, and was 'maddened' by the father's loud voice and contempt for his wife. 'Maddened' thus describes both the therapist's anger and scrambled mind. Struggling to surface, she was startled when Father suddenly said to her: 'Do you know, love ...?'.

The casual use of 'love' to address the therapist seemed to transfer the sexual act and procreation from father and mother to father and her. She experienced it as an intrusion, which was aimed at creating a hostile coupling against the mother. In reflecting later, the therapist considered that Father may have apprehended her 'maddened state' and unconscious alignment with his wife, and responded to this. 'Love' may have therefore been used as a carapace of contempt, an 'anti-analytic third' discourse (Straker, 2006) that compromised the therapist through use of proscribed gendered relations. The debasement of the female object seemed a necessary defence on this father's part against his own madness and disintegration, and – in that moment – precluded reflectiveness. In this case, this pattern did not shift until much later, after the therapy had ended. Father requested a meeting with the therapist to discuss the impact on him and their little boy of yet another prolonged hospitalisation of the mother. It seemed that he came back to the consulting room in search of a benign mothering figure to support his own nurturing qualities towards his child.

Sexuality can also be an important constructive force within the therapy, particularly when it couples the parents protectively around their child. In the case below the sexualised fantasy of a father-to-be was brought fruitfully into the therapeutic work, as it generated a path to unconscious imagery and fantasy around becoming a family.

Father-to-be J joined the therapy in the second session with his pregnant partner, R. The therapist invited J to tell her about himself and quickly learned that J, like R, suffered severe and long-standing mental health problems. Both parents-to-be worried that this increased their vulnerability in the transition to parenthood. There was a moment of reflection after this was stated, and then J broke into a rush of words:

> The baby is going to come and it's going to have all these things to mess with you and screw you over, and all these good things as well, but you've got to try to understand how it's going to screw you over – without meaning to, so that you can develop strategies to deal with that. I'm open minded as to how we deal with its particular needs. I'm ready for the challenge.

The therapist was taken aback by the vehemence in father's voice and words, but also intrigued by his communication. The expressions 'mess with you', 'screw you over' and 'beat the hell out of you' have highly emotive connotations of sexual violation and beating. Whether it was a fantasy of the primal scene, wherein sexual intercourse was perceived as an act of violent aggression on the part of the father whose baby was metaphorically raped into existence and will extract its revenge, or a fantasised transgenerational Oedipal murder, it was clear that these attributions could potentially shape J's experience of his baby (a boy) and relationship with him. Carefully paced therapeutic work enabled substantial unpacking of J's fears. It also facilitated dialogue between him and R, who carried quite different imagery of conception and parenting.

In both this and the previous cases the mother was the referred patient by the professionals, and the fathers were off the professionals' radar, presumably seen as the non-problematic parents. However, in each case the father's personality and defensive systems permitted very different use of parent-infant psychotherapy.. The father who addressed the therapist as 'love' used sexualisation of the relationship with the therapist defensively; in the case of J sexuality and fecundity were brought to the therapy for psychological work. Their partners also brought very different expectancies. In the first case the mother fully identified with her husband's pathologising in a transgenerational identification with a mother as a degraded object. In the latter case, R and J were accustomed to supporting each other through discussion and exploration. Finally, the therapist's countertransference played its role in the trajectory of engagement and treatment. Paternal projections of contempt, expressed in the mismatch between the word 'love' and bodily expression, were difficult to process. J's impulsive torrent evoked surprise, curiosity and empathy. The amalgam of emotions, representations and behaviours in each instance influenced the possibilities for inclusion or exclusion of father in the therapy.

Chapter 8

The male therapist in parent-infant psychotherapy

Abel Fagin

Introduction

In this chapter I make the case that gender impacts upon the course of parent-infant psychotherapy and that the male therapist may have a distinct influence whether there is a father presence or absence. I have chosen to focus my discussion of families where there is significant instability, as I consider the male therapist as having an emblematic role in preserving or modelling the experience of the parental couple and co-parenting relationship when it is at risk. I present two cases of work, one with a mother-father-infant triad and another with a mother-infant dyad, to explore the distinguishing ways in which the male therapist may support a parenting couple and offer a model of a co-parenting experience. The effectiveness of the approach appears to be determined by whether this is felt as a threat, an unremitting hunger for a father or partner presence, or experienced as an alternate paternal male figure who can offer a transformative relationship (Bollas, 1979) through a temporary experience of care.

In my thinking about my work as a male therapist it is not possible to extricate myself from cultural expectations and those that emerge in the field of psychotherapy. These values, beliefs and ideas shape psychological life and the process of my work. As important as it is to acknowledge each family's own gender stories and experiences of fathering, it is also necessary to be aware of the influences from my own personal and professional context, and those values and qualities that I privilege in my work. Although I focus on heterosexual relationships, I would hope this discussion remains of relevance to a range of family set-ups.

I work in predominantly female environments in a profession that is largely female orientated. McHale & Phares (2015) cite research indicating that over 95% of staff who serve families and young children were women and are not as comfortable and accustomed to working with fathers as they are with mothers. I believe this finding indicates an anxiety about men and women working in a closed off or intimate setting, and although it centres on the experiences of female staff working with fathers, it does not seem far-fetched to imagine that there are similar anxieties present which influence the work with a male therapist and their colleagues and clients. Further, as it is less conventional for males to train in this specialist area, perhaps this novelty has fuelled the occasional curiosity and suspicion I have encountered.

I believe it is important to consider how the attributions from colleagues and clients towards my male gender may start to influence the course of therapeutic work. I have had experience of colleagues who have presuppositions about whether, as a man, it is appropriate for me to take on work with a particular family. While offering a choice of male or female therapist is commonplace in all therapeutic domains, I do believe there is some bias towards mothers being given the choice as to whether they wish to meet with me or not and they are often asked if they are comfortable working with a man. Perhaps to some degree this parallels the view that fathers are less important or viewed as a 'third wheel', as excluded from the developing relationship between mother and baby. There are some families where this is appropriate on cultural and religious grounds, but in other cases it may disregard the value of the infant developing within a triangular structure. It may also create a sense of uncertainty about the risks that men might pose and potentially conveys a view that this option is a second choice. Reflections on these biases, often not spoken about within a team or with referrers, can shape how families are considered for treatment in a way that does not act upon on fears that might hinder therapeutic change, but create openings to address gender-related sources of difficulty.

To some degree these general anxieties about a male therapist working with vulnerable families in the perinatal period appear to relate to whether I can sufficiently identify with nurturing and protective maternal qualities. As an extreme it suggests a phantasy that I risk repeating previous traumas, such as succumbing to an innate primitive aggression or sexual urge. This can perpetuate the view of a male as a predatory figure, and positions the male as the active sexual being and the female as passive. From the patient's point of view, it goes without saying that there are indeed mothers who are unsure whether men can be trusted or can understand the experience of motherhood. It does not mean that therapy with a male therapist cannot progress if they are not too overwhelmed by this prospect.

It is also the case that fathers too may feel uneasy working with male therapists, who may worry about becoming emasculated through emotional disclosure, intimacy and dependence. I recall a father in an assessment saying 'I'm happy that I just have that time when I come back at the end of the day, I couldn't deal with looking after him [baby] all day.' It seemed that 'the end of the day' was all this man could tolerate in terms of his baby's dependency. Fathers may also feel threatened by being displaced by the male therapist, fearing this intruder may disempower him or capture the heart of his partner and child. One may wonder what fantasies arise when a father chooses not to attend, and whether this fuels feelings of exclusion. Often there is a discussion of the risks associated with female parent-infant psychotherapist being positioned as a better mother. Perhaps the male parent-infant psychotherapist also risks being in a position of a better father or partner.

Gender is a definitive marker the therapist brings into the room. Gender and the erotic cannot be removed from the psychically binding relationships and are mediums through which transformation can occur. In this context, the male therapist may reflect upon the gender-related wishes, fantasies and transferences which arise in the work and may be challenged by how multiple transferential relationships touch upon the therapist's own internal world and unconscious wishes from the therapeutic encounter. I hope that the following discussion will enable insights into the process of parent-infant psychotherapy with a male therapist.

Setting the scene

Dugmore (2014) highlights how the 'flexing' of the frame in parent-infant psychotherapy is a necessary adaption to engage multiple family members while attempting to maintain 'psychoanalytic mindfulness' to limit enactments. In parent-infant psychotherapy, the therapist is often mobile and responsive to the shifting demands in the room and thus thrown into being immersed and exposed to dynamics which limit a capacity to remain 'mindful'. The physical space shared between each participant is likely to influence the experience of each configuration, such as shifting between dyadic and triadic work, where some members may be included or excluded. The setting often requests that each member arrange themselves so as to be able to make contact with the infant, opening up the forum to explore the relationship configurations, and also bringing parental and gender identifications to the fore. For example, the male therapist may find himself aligning with the mother-infant relationship which may reignite Oedipal anxieties and feelings of exclusion.

Parent-infant psychotherapy imposes degrees of increased intimacy which are likely to be experienced differently with a male therapist. Physical distance and boundaries are maintained in the degree of contact the therapist has with the parents, although this is often not the case for how the therapist relates to the infant. The therapist is an active participant and is typically open to foster, scaffold and model a nurturing, creative and playful relationship with the infant. In a way which is child-led and facilitating for the infant, the therapist may initiate and receive appropriate touch, exploration and closeness to take place. In caring for the infant in a developmentally sensitive manner, the male therapist not only provides a facilitating environment for the baby, but also may elicit memories and absences of the parents' own experiences of being parented by a male and consequently open up future possibilities of how male care is offered.

Working with the triad

Having a baby can increase the risk of relationship breakdown in all individuals, and these risks increase with those who have experienced degrees of early deprivation and trauma in the family environment, particularly those who have not had the opportunity to establish their couple relationship and prepare for having a baby (Galdiolo & Roskan, 2016). Helping to manage the impact of past trauma, absence or conflict without harmfully impinging on the baby can be a focal area of parent-infant work. While the above are tasks of any parent-infant psychotherapist, what difference does it make if this is by a man or a woman?

This may largely depend on how the male therapist impacts upon each individual's capacity to hold the co-parenting relationship in mind, as past and present conflicts and transferential dynamics come to the fore. Feelings of exclusion and displacement are commonly reported by new parents, especially fathers, who have been characterised as not only being excluded from the developing relationship between mother and baby but also from the intimate and sexual relationship with the mother before the birth.

The male therapist communicating that he both values the evolving nature of the father-baby relationship and is able to hold the 'couple state of mind' (Morgan, 2001) can reinforce respect for father's position of importance and limit the perception that he is someone who may take over, intrude or compete. He not only offers an alternate parental presence, but confounds the view of him as a rival. Supporting the father to claim his baby and reclaim his relationship with his partner requires the male therapist to attend to the tie between mother and baby, where some mothers may feel that their maternal role is threatened by a father's wish to become more involved. These anxieties may be heightened if there is not sufficient safety to explore these experiences and accommodate changes in parental functioning and it may also feel that there is a monopolising alliance between father and male therapist. Moreover, there is often a pull towards forming an alliance with one particular member, or viewing the infant only in terms of his or her dyadic rather than triadic experiences. This may be indicative of the parental couple being unable to take a third position (Britton, 1989) where there may be defensive responses to making links and reflection. This can be influenced by the gendered experience of the transference, for example, if the male presence elicits memories or enactments from the past which inhibit or facilitate opportunities to mentalise.

Ideally, observing and reflecting upon the shared experience of the couple relationship with their baby can help them both to feel more included and creates a therapeutic environment which can help them process and understand conflict, rather than it being carried out as an enactment. By working to preserve the parental couple (where this is possible), Oedipal anxieties in the parents can be addressed, which supports the parents' ability to offer their infant an experience of joint thinking and co-operation.

Example: Tayo, Sade and Enofe

I present the following example of father Tayo, mother Sade and baby Enofe, with whom I began working during the pregnancy. The couple were a 'love marriage', which was against their parent's traditional values and caused them to become estranged from the wider network. Tayo's father was physically abusive and violent, and Tayo had tried to end his life in his adolescence. Although Sade described her upbringing as more stable, it was highly upsetting when her family severed their support after her marriage. The couple had lived comfortably in the UK until faced with a series of events related to their work and immigration status that changed their lives. Because of their circumstances, Sade reluctantly had an abortion, which caused significant distress. In this second pregnancy she became depressed and felt detached from the baby, fearing that something bad would happen. Tayo could not imagine himself caring for a baby, and felt that he had failed his family. The experience of failure and loss seemed to consume them both individually and communication between them suffered terribly.

The work focused on the therapist assisting the parental couple to explore the impact of personal loss and trauma, and how feelings of helplessness influenced their feeling isolated from each other. Offering a benign paternal presence and modelling a male representation of care seemed to reframe Tayo's view of emotional disclosure and sensitivity as a weakness, and supported his wish to challenge the familial and cultural expectations of him as the ancillary parent. It was important to make a distinction between Tayo's lack of protection as a child and the current beliefs about not being able to protect and provide for his family. We were able to identify how this felt like a repetition of Tayo's earlier experiences of uncertainty and a threatening environment. In the therapeutic space, the couple were able to imagine the impact of their shared difficulties on Enofe and came together to offer an experience of nurturing care. While feeling a sense of failure because they were not being able to provide him with the material goods they would have wished for, they were united in the value that their love had for him.

In the above example, it was possible to work directly with both parents to preserve the couple relationship, and to help the father develop an alternate view of himself as an effective parent. When the father does not attend in therapy but remains in a partnership or caregiving role, the male therapist continues to keep the couple in mind. For example, in a situation where a mother might convey her unhappiness in the parental relationship, the male therapist might seek to attend to both her experience and her understanding of the father's and the child's experiences in order to explore how the couple might co-parent their child.

As not all relationships are able to be preserved, the male therapist may be placed in a position where he is called on to offer a reparative male and fatherly presence.

The challenges of becoming a reparative male figure

Relationship breakdowns in the perinatal period are a crisis for mother, father and baby, but fathers are at greatest risk of exclusion. Mothers are commonly viewed as the gateway to the baby, both in terms of physical access to the baby and symbolically. She will significantly influence how the father and their couple relationship is portrayed to her baby. This is likely to be influenced by her representation of the father of the child and the breakdown of their relationship as well as her representations of men and the fatherly role. Mothers may experience doubt as to whether they might be able to foster future intimate relationships and if these might be harmful to their baby. They may become overly self-reliant in the attempt to shut off from the feelings about the baby's conception or dissolved relationship. There are also some who find feelings of anger, loneliness and abandonment unbearable. All these factors will affect the access the father has to his child and whether he can mitigate the mother's negative representations.

If couple relationships do end in separation, it is most common that parent-infant work occurs with the mother and baby alone. Although there may have been attempts to do this, it often means that the father's position has not been explored with him and the mother to make sense of what has occurred in their family life and how they may plan as co-parents.

When there is an acrimonious split in the relationship, as a male therapist there is a danger of further magnifying the split between a good (available and understanding therapist) and bad (absent) father. This may limit how these relationships are thought about and integrated. When the split results in the father absenting himself from therapy, there is inevitably the creation of an alternate relationship with a man (therapist) which may consequently reinforce the displacement of the father. Without an attempt to keep past experiences of fathering and the father's position as part of the work, it may be experienced as 'killing him off'. It is important to shift investment in the therapist becoming a replacement and to communicate the reality of his position. The therapist will then need to address the dynamics which arise in mother-infant work with a male that construct a relational template of a father/partner presence as a model of a co-parenting relationship, rather than affirming an illusion that he can completely fulfil that role.

Participation in therapy with a man may take a different course with respect to preventing premature flights into new relationships. Optimally, the therapy relies on the mother permitting alternate, reparative relationships to form in order to facilitate the reworking of previous representations. It is the hope that this creates a more flexible representation of a co-parenting partnership in her mind and that this can be conveyed to her baby. In doing so, the quality of this partnership may enable the male therapist greater flexibility in his provision of care and alter the way in which father figures are thought about.

There are a number of dilemmas I have encountered in achieving this. An experience of a benign male figure is presented but may be guarded against because of an uncertainty that further harm will be perpetrated by a male figure and the therapy (ab)used to lull the mother into a false sense of security. The male therapist is likely to be prone to transferential processes which seek to confirm or test out whether this is the case. The mother may also be guarded because of an attempt to manage feelings of anger, loss and disappointment linked in to the therapist becoming the fantasised and wished for object. While the male therapist may offer a fatherly presence, he does not provide the level of contact and intimacy that might be wanted.

The mother may face a doubly difficult task of resolving these feelings for herself, and assisting her baby who is developing a representation of how the therapist sits within their relational configuration. The baby is likely to experience the father's absence and yearn to make a connection with this missing object while the therapist is also becoming a significant other. Without sufficient parental resolve, it seems likely that the baby may attempt to understand whether the therapist is indeed the absent father. While it is feasible to explore this distinction with the mother, it is very difficult to do so with an infant. Indeed in my longer-term work, this wish has been expressed verbally by children who have referred to me as 'Daddy'. This situation can result in dilemmas about reigniting earlier losses for both mother and baby.

Yearnings for a partner

Following a break-up, the mother's attachment and sexual intimacy needs for adult relationships are likely to be triggered and manifest in the therapeutic encounter. This may be driven by a need to complement and support her parenting and secure a father presence for her child. There may be a yearning in a mother for an intimate and sexual relationship and this may impact upon her transference to the male therapist and her child's experience of him. The mother may not be only seeking to repair earlier losses but may also be looking for new adult relationships that can offer a different and transformative experience.

It has been long understood that an important contribution to healthy infant development arises out of the appropriate investment of the mother's libido in the baby and the excitation of the baby's erogenous zones (Freud, 1905). What seems to be largely missing from the literature is how the mother's libido changes postnatally, and especially when loss of the partner may stimulate sexual phantasies and partner seeking, and how this may impact the baby. Ignoring this aspect in mother and infant relationships may in part be an effort to desexualise the mother's needs for fear that the erotic may pose a threat to the infant (Mann, 1999). There is a danger that failing to pick up on eroticised feelings may further perpetuate fears around sexual desire and wishing for a relationship, and the therapist may become identified with an emotionally unavailable object. In such circumstances, he may find that he contributes to enmeshment if the mother turns to her baby to meet these needs. It therefore becomes more important to attend to the transference when the mother's eroticisation of the relationship with the baby is a defence against the yearnings towards the therapist.

Perinatal relationship breakdown is likely to evoke earlier losses and unrequited longings from childhood. Herzog (2014) describes a 'father hunger' as a child's yearning for the father who can be receptive to contain and modulate the child's aggressive drives and fantasies, and also plays a significant role in intruding upon the mother-infant symbiosis. It is important to consider the degree to which the mother's longings for a male figure shift the focus away from the therapeutic relationship and parent-infant relationship. Yet, it also may be the case that there is a window of opportunity to address past and present losses with another male, albeit in a more limited way, while these are more accessible. This can assist in developing mother and infant's sense of agency in being able to claim and recruit another's personal investment in them which might provide an opportunity to both support and open up a port of entry into their relationship.

The infant's interest in the therapist is likely to be facilitated by the therapist's wishes to foster an environment which promotes understanding, communication, creative growth and care but also when appropriate to take up elements of parenting to compliment and aid the parent where necessary. These may be co-constructed as arising from the male therapist's own qualities and experience of being parented, and also those enacted from unconscious wishes and yearnings by the patient. This may have, or be perceived as having, a male or paternal quality (e.g. extending episodes of play or regulating mother and baby).

The infant's gender may also significantly influence the parents' experience of the infant in relation with the male therapist. I have encountered mothers who, without the presence of a father, come to heavily invest in the relationship with their infant sons in a manner which seeks to compensate for their loss. If there is sufficient openness to this encounter, the male therapist may have a role in drawing the infant away from mother and offer an array of interaction that is not confined to fulfilling the mother's wishes for an adult relationship. The infant may be interested in having different experiences to the ones shared with mother and offers a potential opportunity to experience a couple who is invested in him. Being open to this allows the infant to explore this relationship and alternate figure intimately, allowing the development of curiosity, closeness and an experience of security. The male therapist may also offer respite to the infant during periods where the mother is overwhelmed and provide an opportunity for mother and baby to re-connect when she is more able. This also creates an experience and develops a representation in the mother's mind of the infant being cared for by an alternate male other. The mother may also identify with their infant's experience, which can be effective when the infant is seen in their own right, but may also evoke confusing feelings. These can arise if the mother becomes envious of the contact the therapist shares with the baby as she cannot receive the physical presence and intimacy that her baby is eligible to.

The mother's yearning for a partner in combination with the infant's developing relationship with the male therapist may contribute to a formation of a parental couple and link in the mother's mind. Conflicts can arise when this psychological coupling cannot happen in reality. This wish may not only be driven to find a sufficient replacement for the loss of father, but also may represent longings for her own absent father and incestual Oedipal desire. This often does not arise within the therapeutic dialogue but can be powerfully expressed by both mother and baby through a sexualised transference as well as attraction or sexual feelings arising in the counter transference. However, feelings of love and sexual feelings may be part of a transformational and creative process and not necessarily a therapeutic impasse (Mann, 1999). The therapeutic endeavour is one which involves a creative pursuit and the male therapist may be perceived as offering a potency through the investment in this work. Mann (ibid.) suggests that the therapeutic endeavour is a symbolic intercourse which has the potential to conceive and give birth to new ideas and psychic change. The degree by which erotic feelings become part of the psychic link between individuals needs to be managed but should not be denied as these feelings might signify a process in which the mother becomes more open to the presence of the male therapist and the relationship they can have with their child.

I strive to remain curious about these experiences, and through self-reflection and supervision, seek to process uncomfortable feelings such as attraction, guilt and anxiety when they arise. In the therapeutic encounter, sometimes speaking about these directly is unhelpful and may be experienced as a provocation or seduction, but being able to contain them and be open to these feelings will be of significance to the client. On the other hand, with some patients it is possible to explore the expectations, disappointment and limitations of the therapeutic role in a sensitive and boundaried way. The challenge lies in whether these feelings are held rigidly and acted on as a reality, or whether the loss can be reflected on in the context of the situation.

I would like to present an example of work with a mother and daughter where I felt a considerable personal investment in the family. This was tied to my efforts to maintain the therapeutic alliance with the parent because of the risks posed to the infant. There were high levels of anxiety relating to the parent disengaging and concern not only about the loss of a protective role of the therapist, but also the absence of a figure who had become a significant, alternative and nurturing other to the infant. The father had chosen to not remain part of their family life and also presented a risk of violence.

Example: Katriya and Sophie

I was playing with Sophie (18 months) sharing toy food while her mother was looking affectionately on. Sophie moved closer to me and snuggled into my lap and we continued to play. She got up and walked towards her mother, and looked up at her. She looked at me coyly and hesitated. She then pursed her lips and came forward and kissed me. Her mother looked a little surprised and laughed in a way which indicated some discomfort. She called her daughter's name out in a way which both supported and condoned her behaviour. Katriya appeared to emotionally withdraw, and said dismissively that she does this with all the men she sees. Katriya put her hands out and called out asking for a kiss, but Sophie turned away. A few moments later, Katriya asked again for a kiss and moved towards her, bringing her closer to make contact. Sophie turned her head and her mother's face stilled with resentment and frustration. The atmosphere became tense and unpredictable, and I sensed Katriya's anger and rejection. I could not make out if she was letting her daughter go or whether she was pushing her away.

At this time, it was rare that Sophie sought affection from her mother and this may have felt like a repetition of how others rejected Katriya in her past. While she wished her daughter to have a different experience from her own neglect, she became envious, severing and denigrating the links which were emerging. Perhaps she was feeling under threat from my role of significant male other and how I may act as penetrating her symbiotic reliance on her daughter. Sophia had greater flexibility in being able to be coy and flirtatious with me, while mother could not. I had felt that this was an intimate moment between us all. It may have been the case that Sophia was expressing her mother's desires, possibly acting upon Katriya's eroticised feelings that were projected into her.

Katriya is envious of the 'love' I receive and who I might represent as a father figure that she yearned for. She calls for her own kiss but Sophia turns away leading to feelings of humiliation and fury with myself as well as her daughter. Katriya struggled to acknowledge her desperate need for a relationship, and her defensive responses were carried out in a forceful and attacking manner, and resulted in repeated experience of loneliness and rejection.

One may wonder if the quality of the paternal function changes according to the gender of therapist, and I believe that this depends upon the meaning that this has to the individual and what is evoked in the transference. The degree to which parents show concern for their infant and can sufficiently trust and be receptive to the presence of a third who is able to regulate and penetrate a psychologically compromised caregiving relationship will likely be a key factor in beneficial outcomes. In the early stages of work, Katriya did not have a representation of parental co-operation and likely saw male figures, such as myself, with considerable suspicion. It seemed my role as therapist was to mop up Katriya's anger and provide Sophie with a period of respite during our time together. I was concerned about the volatility of the parent-infant relationship and whether progress could be made.

I often felt flooded by Katriya which prevented me from engaging with Sophie and left me feeling impotent and frustrated. She denied the links I would make around my significance and the progress we had made in the work, communicating that others could not be helpful. I understood my feelings as being located in her experience of unsuccessful attempts to find care from emotionally unavailable parents and the lack of love, mistrust and co-operation between them. She blamed her father and also harboured considerable rage towards Sophie's father as well as guilt and failure about their relationship ending, primarily because she did not foresee his abusive behaviour and this confirmed her beliefs about untrustworthy men.

I believe there were critical moments of becoming a parental couple in mind which conveyed my efforts to nurture and protect rather than perpetuate a pattern of male relationships which were abusive. It was important to understand Katriya's rage and helplessness, even when I felt that this was an expression of her need to get closer. I needed to create a sense of safety by holding onto the conscious and unconscious parts of her and to not repeat harmful situations such as impulsively responding to my frustration and need to shield Sophie. She began to permit a space to acknowledge her anger and in turn facilitated an awareness of how her hostility impacted on Sophie. It gave rise to helping her with feelings of guilt and a wish to repair the effects of earlier turmoil. She was more able to identify as a protective figure and was less envious that Sophie could experience nurturance, as well as a different relationship with myself, that she did not receive herself.

Katriya started to see me as a male that was available to her that could contain her destructiveness and not abandon her. Nevertheless, I believe she kept on her guard because I could not fulfil her wishes of becoming her partner and Sophie's father. This communicated that loss and disappointment could be experienced but did not lead to separation and disarray. There was a shared investment by both mother and myself, which despite the limitations, may have offered Sophie an experience of her mother and a male in alliance. This appears to have created a transformational experience with a male which hopefully helped to heal the past and perhaps the future.

Summary

This chapter highlights how the male therapist may have a distinct influence in parent-infant psychotherapy where there is a father presence as well as an absence. The male therapist has a distinct role in preserving the parental couple when the father is present, and where he is absent, he might offer the experience of the parental couple and co-parenting relationship. It has been discussed how this is determined by the transference and whether there are enough opportunities to be experienced as an alternate male figure within the limitations of the therapeutic work.

I have also highlighted the importance of acknowledging gender in the therapeutic work and how erotic feelings are likely to be common place.

Sexual feelings occurring in parent-infant psychotherapy have not received sufficient attention. This may have created a context where these are experienced as taboo. This is possibly connected with, and perhaps more so in the case of a male therapist, fears of abusive practice. This has implications for the therapist's own reflection and how it is thought about, or not, in the supervisory space, and furthermore, whether the gender of the supervisor is also of significance.

Since gender does, in my view, impact upon the course of parent-infant psychotherapy there is also a space in the literature for a critical examination of how women may influence the therapeutic process, particularly in their work with fathers.

Chapter 9

The therapist and the father in parent-infant psychotherapy

Yael Segal

Clinical experience has shown that fathers attend parent-infant psychotherapy less frequently than their partners, and when they do it is usually at the therapist's request. Even then, the father usually joins in for only a limited number of sessions. This may be due to factors residing with the father, the mother or the therapist. For example, the father may object to therapy based on his social-cultural values or due to defences or difficulty accepting help. The mother may wish to distance the father from her bond with the baby and/or the therapist, or may be afraid to expose negative thoughts and feelings in his presence. And the therapist may be held back by her countertransference. It is on the latter that I will focus in this chapter. I will suggest that a negative countertransference can raise an unconscious resistance in the therapist to the father's participation in the therapy, contrary to her declared positive attitude. I will discuss two types of resistance and their resolution: *cultural bias* and *the father as a man.*

Cultural bias

Infant caregiving, which is heavily loaded with values, conceptions and preconceptions formed by thousands of years of human evolution, puts the mother-infant relationship squarely at the centre.

> No complicated society with a written tradition has ever expected the man of stature and education to care for a baby. Mothers, nurses, female relatives, children, even eunuchs, but not fathers, had the physical care of young infants. So it has been possible to say that there seemed to be no instinctive basis for fatherhood comparable to the instinctive basis of maternal behaviour.
>
> (Mead, 1957, p. 374)

Notions of gender equality among therapists, as in general society, are relatively new, and the tendency to prioritise the exclusive mother-infant relationship has deep roots in our culture, finding expression even in the clinical psychoanalytic theories by which most of our therapists are trained.

The assimilation of new ideas into clinical theory and practice takes more time than it does to formulate them. Even theories about the importance of the mother-infant relationship for individual development needed time to mature and to find expression in clinical practice, as in the case of attachment theory. But the important formulations provided by psychoanalysts, which psychotherapists could rely upon as a frame and 'compass' and use as guidelines to understanding subjective experience and the dynamics of transference in their clinical work, remained limited to the mother-infant relationship. Such, for example, was Winnicott's formulation of 'primary maternal preoccupation' (Winnicott, 1956) and Stern's 'motherhood constellation' (Stern, 1995).

The novelty in Winnicott and Stern's formulations was to define the psychic state of the newborn baby's mother as exclusively and transiently experienced immediately after birth – neither before nor later in life. For Winnicott:

> primary maternal preoccupation is a very special state of the mother ... an organized psychological condition in which some aspect of the personality takes over temporarily ... she must be able to reach this state of heightened sensitivity, almost an illness ... and to recover from it.
>
> (Winnicott, 1956, p. 302)

> Mothers become able in a specialized way to step into the shoes of the baby ... to almost lose themselves in an identification with the baby so they know what the baby needs at this very moment.
>
> (Winnicott, 1949, p. 94)

Stern (1995) stated that the 'motherhood constellation' was a unique psychic organisation that emerged in the mother with the birth of a baby, especially her first-born. It determined a new set of action tendencies, sensibilities, fantasies, fears and wishes, and became the dominant organising axis of the mother's psychic life. It pushed aside the previous nuclear organisations that played a central role, and her preoccupations now became centred on the grandmother-mother-baby triad. Such formulations are enormously helpful in parent-infant clinical practice because they force clinicians to adopt a new therapeutic stance. Without an appreciation of the nature and predominance of the psychic organisation they describe, it would be difficult to grasp the main subjective themes that mothers experience, the shape of the problems for which they seek help, and especially the form of the transference they develop.

According to Winnicott and Stern, fathers can be good caregivers, but they do not experience the particular psychic state that mothers do. This idea receives support from recent brain research showing that the psychic state governing the father's caregiving activity arrives through different brain-pathways than that of the mother: mothers showed greater activation in the emotional processing network and fathers in the socio-cognitive circuits (Abraham et al., 2014b). This is not a devaluation of the father. What I wish to emphasise is rather the lack of a complementary 'fatherhood constellation' for understanding the subjective experience of the father of a newborn baby, for I believe that fathers, like mothers, also experience a unique psychic organisation for some time after their child's birth. Such a formulation is a necessary guide in clinical parent-infant work, especially for understanding the father's needs as they become manifested in the transference.

The marginal attention paid by Stern and Winnicott to the father, who is mainly allocated the task of supporting the mother, has been duly addressed in the professional literature, and it is not my intention to enlarge on it further. This chapter addresses the lack of a theoretical formulation of the new father's subjective experience. Accumulated clinical experience shows that following the birth of a child, not only the woman but the man, too, undergoes a profound developmental change in his transition from manhood into fatherhood. He too develops a unique psychic organisation deserving the name of 'fatherhood constellation', which differs from the mother's and can provide clinicians with specific theoretical guidelines. In my view, the main factor that is unique to the new father's psychic constellation is the threat posed to his manhood. Therapists often miss how much the birth of a baby can undermine the father's male identity.

Every person's earliest identification is with the mother figure (Stoller, 1994). Yet while this identification has continuity in the psychic life of the girl, the boy who is beginning to establish his male identity must make the necessary and appropriate break away from his primary identification with his mother. In the success of this break the mother plays a major role. If she enables and encourages the appropriate disidentification from her, the boy stands a good chance of completing the process optimally. However, if she opposes it for various reasons, such as her own difficulty separating or her hostile emotions towards male figures, then her son's male identity will henceforth remain vulnerable, and any feminine and maternal traits will be associated in his mind with submissiveness and fear of the tyrannical or seductive female. His male identity will therefore always be threatened by women or by femininity in himself or in others.

The birth of a baby arouses in both parents the need to respond to it and to care for it in a manner that is considered maternal, so that in both mother and father an early, primary identification instinctively arises with the mother who cared for them in infancy. Yet while a direct, continuous line connects the mother of the present with her own mother in infancy through this identification, in the father there is a conflicted and potentially vulnerable area because of the way the male identity became established. When the baby is born, the father's male identity comes under strain, and the outcome of this phase depends on the way he deals with the reawakening inside him of the maternal and female aspects of his own identity as a caregiver, or of the baby he once was. Will these aspects find a place in his new identity as a man and father?

If the early process of breaking away followed a healthy and normal course and his male identity was satisfactorily established in his childhood, the new father will show aspects of good mothering in his parental role. However, if the mother figure remains a threat to his manhood, we will see it in the transference in the form of avoidance, anxiety or sexualisation common reactions designed to ward off the reawakening of feelings of dependency and the threat to his psychic autonomy.

In the absence of a 'fatherhood constellation' to help therapists understand this dynamic, their work with fathers is at risk of being less organised and of shifting uneasily between an ordinary psychodynamic attitude that fails to take the fatherhood constellation into consideration, and one that is simply confused and inconsistent. This can create in the therapy an area that is overly affected by the therapist's unconscious countertransference reactions. The patient may represent for the analyst an object of the past on to whom past feelings and wishes are projected. The analyst's countertransference may also be part of the patient's personality and past object relationships, the patient's 'creation' in the transference. If not identified as such, it can harm her empathic ability; but if she 'reads the map', the counter-transference can be reversed from being an interference to becoming a potential source of vital confirmation (Racker, 1982). A distinction should be made between 'personal countertransference', which has to do with the therapist, and a 'diagnostic countertransference' that indicates something about the patient. The therapist must be able to tell the difference between cases in which her reactions to the patient are telling her something about his psychic state, and those in which they are merely expressing hers. When she fails, her ability to be fully attentive to her patient is compromised.

To summarise, psychotherapists who are not equipped with satisfactory theoretical guidelines for understanding fathers will be less controlled and more subject to the personal, cultural and sociological biases of their unconscious and non-conscious attitudes towards men, and these will inevitably find expression in the countertransference. When a therapist's cultural biases combine with her early object relations, it is evident how, unconsciously, the results will be re-enacted in the therapy. It then requires great effort to resolve and counteract the deep-seated inclination to prioritise the mother-infant relationship, and make room for the father.

Clinical case

Anna, mother of Danny, age two months, was referred because of Danny's frequent vomiting, up to five or six times a day. Reflux was ruled out and the doctor said he was being overfed. Anna denied this, saying it was impossible because Danny was exclusively breastfed. At the first session the therapist was impressed by the mother's high level of anxiety. Anna said that her mother's anxiety since her father's death two years ago was contagious and that she constantly had to calm her down. In fact, the entire family was in a perpetual state of anxiety. Anna's father had held the family together, and in his absence things were falling apart and there was no one to reassure them. Danny too seemed anxious and tense, clinging to his mother with his gaze. The therapist suggested a connection between Anna's anxiety and the infant's vomiting as an expression of the anxiety he had caught from her. She accepted the interpretation immediately, wondering how she hadn't thought of such an obvious explanation herself. She said that with his father Danny was better; he smiled and was more relaxed. She added that her husband took over whenever she felt resentful and disconnected from Danny. But he criticised her mothering bitterly. He thought she was stuffing Danny and that she was overanxious to the point of being unbearable. Anna admitted that she fed Danny even in the absence of any signs of hunger, feeling it was the only way she knew how to calm him. Eventually, watching their interaction, it became clear that although she was able to read Danny accurately and understand the meaning of his cues, she could not respond in accordance with his needs. Anna said she had not been understood as a child because she used to hide her true feelings, and now she was afraid she would miss her baby's actual condition. In the following sessions her fear of death (her own and her baby's) emerged more clearly. It had first appeared after her father's death, and reached its peak during her labour with Danny. She felt near death at the time, because her pains were so severe and her fever so high that she lost consciousness several times and was delirious. She was sure she was dying, and this fear was transferred to Danny. Now she was afraid he wouldn't survive unless she fed him, and only feeding him would calm her fear. It was only at this point that the father was invited to join the therapy, in order to help in the reconstruction of the traumatic labour. She had forgotten most of it. She doubted whether he would come because of his military service far from home and his unwillingness to talk. She was wrong.

The father, handsome and impressive in his officer's uniform, came in and brought into the room a wave of strong manhood, with the unmistakable smell of military laundry. He spoke easily, despite signs of embarrassment, such as refusing to take off his shoes. To the mother's and therapist's surprise, he said he liked to talk and wanted to answer the therapist's questions. Danny smiled when interacting with him and was more relaxed than with his mother. When they spoke about the labour, he argued with Anna defensively, saying it hadn't been as bad as she made it out to be, but agreed to reconstruct it with her. The recollection of the suppressed details was very meaningful to her, giving the traumatic event a different and more optimistic ending that all three of them could share in some happy moments at the end of the session.

In the following session the father mentioned he likes talking about these things. But since Danny was now showing dramatic developmental progress, the therapist concluded that the father need not be disturbed any further, and he was left out of the therapy. In retrospect it seems clear that the two sessions with the father were a turning point in the therapy, which should have continued in its triadic mother-father-baby setting. But the therapist, blind to these dynamics, failed to use the opportunity and dropped the father whom she considered a temporary and no longer necessary 'co-therapist' in her work with the mother. The treatment ended a few months later, with the relationship between mother and baby warm and pleasurable and Danny's development proceeding on a normal track. In the final session Anna told the therapist how happy she felt with Danny and how pleased she was with his development. There was only one thing disturbing this situation, and this was the father. Anna felt he was jealous of her closeness to Danny and frustrated because his own relationship with Danny was no longer as good as it used to be. Again, the therapist, happy with the good results, ignored these warning signals.

When Danny was two years old Anna called and told the therapist that although she had been greatly helped by the therapy and was happy with Danny, the relationship between father and son had deteriorated since the end of the treatment. Her husband was no longer the good father he used to be, and he had become jealous of Danny's love for her. He was angry and impatient with Danny, and Danny avoided him and sometimes even seemed frightened of him. Anna said that although he denied it, she thought her husband was suffering from depression ever since Danny's birth. The therapist, remembering how the therapy ended, realised that it had been premature, and that the exclusion of the father had left the triad in a state of imbalance. She asked Anna to invite her husband back into therapy. Anna doubted he would come, but again she was wrong.

He came willingly, saying that he liked to come and talk, but he made it clear that he wasn't interested in making any changes in himself. The therapist suggested that the aim of the therapy would not be to change him but to allow him a better understanding of his son. Based on this agreement they resumed a father-infant psychotherapy. The work followed the usual guidelines for parent-infant therapy: reflecting on their interactions, dealing with the father's ghosts from the past, and profiting from the therapist's modelling, guidance and mirroring. The therapy reached a natural ending when the relationship between father and son became more relaxed and pleasurable for both of them.

How could an experienced therapist be so blind to the father's obvious need and wish to be her patient? The answer, clues to which could be found in her countertransference response, was discovered in her self-analysis. Her own father, an admired military officer who was absent most of her childhood, had been sent on a nine-month mission when she was only a month old. When she became a mother herself she asked her mother how she could accept her husband leaving her for so long, and she had replied, 'In those days men serving the country had to do what they were ordered ... Anyway, it wasn't so bad. I went to live with your grandma and it was very convenient.' Danny's impressive father had aroused the therapist's unconscious representations of her father as an admired-but-absent figure and unnecessary caregiver during infancy. The appearance of the patient/

father also evoked the chain of intergenerational transmission in her, whereby she had internalised her own mother's representations of a father/husband who is neither present nor necessary for raising an infant, since the important relationship is grandmother-mother-baby. Fathers were excluded.

The therapist was also denying the impact on the father of the traumatic birth. The reconstruction had been carried out for the mother's benefit, and signs of the father's defensive denial had been ignored. It was only much later that Anna could reflect and say she thought her husband was depressed since Danny was born. Her attitude agreed with the therapist's unconscious representation of the father as a 'brave military man' who never needs any help. This case demonstrates how cultural values can combine with the therapist's personal history to become unconsciously enacted in the form of a blinding countertransference response in the therapy.

The father as a man

The appearance of the father in parent-infant psychotherapy can introduce sexual tension, be it the erotic component in the couple's relationship or sexual tension between father and therapist. This tension can arouse emotions in the therapist that were absent from her relationship with the mother. The father's erotic feelings towards her, if not dealt with by the therapist, can undermine the therapeutic setting, and they require of her an internal reorganisation as well as a thorough understanding of the father's underlying non-sexual needs which have been transformed into sexualisation. However, since the process is occurring in a setting that is not the father's individual psychotherapy, it is harder for therapists to deal with. The baby, as a third and witness, adds to the embarrassment. In individual therapy, the transference-the patient's attitude towards the therapist-is an important source of information for understanding the patient's inner world. In parent-infant therapy, however, analysis of the transference is necessary only insofar as it can help improve the relationship between parent and baby, and therefore it is more limited in nature. Working on the father's sexual feelings towards the therapist in the baby's presence as a witness and third is not suitable for parent-baby therapy, just as the room where the parents' sexual intercourse takes place should be closed to the baby.

The setting in parent-infant psychotherapy has the additional difficulty of permitting and indeed focusing on the non-verbal communication evoked by the less rigidly regimented physical proximity afforded by the playroom, which includes, for example, taking off shoes. The unconscious and nonconscious cues that constitute the nonverbal communication between therapist, parent and baby involve what has loosely been called the 'fast' brain system, as opposed to the 'slow' system. While the 'slow' system allows for conscious reflection and appraisal, the 'fast' system operates outside of conscious awareness, processing non-verbal embodied information at such a rate that the ensuing rapid cueing and responses leave no time for explicit verbal translation or modification in the moment (Lyons-Ruth, 1998). In the case of sexual contents, the therapist has less conscious control over her emotional responses than might be desired, and she must rely heavily on her professional training and self-analysis. The following case demonstrates this phenomenon, which nearly brought the therapy to a premature end.

Clinical case

This case will describe how a father's transference-love aroused an intense negative emotional reaction in the therapist.

Mr O, Eli's father, was referred to our clinic shortly after Eli's birth. Eli's mother was diagnosed with schizophrenia and was allowed to see her son only once a week under supervision of a social worker. The social services, questioning the father's parental competence, required Mr O to accept treatment at our clinic. He was very cooperative, perhaps too much so; his eagerness for the therapeutic relationship became increasingly disturbing to the therapist. After two months of treatment, the therapist began to feel that Mr O wanted her to replace his sick wife. His overt gratitude hardly concealed his erotic feelings. He texted her long poetic messages expressing his infatuation and loaded with erotic allusions. Once he bought her an expensive Parker pen, which she found unable either to accept or reject, seeing it as a barely disguised phallic symbol. In the sessions he 'behaved himself', but she felt embarrassed by his tender looks. Although she understood his behaviour as transference and her aversion as negative counter-transference, she felt sexually harassed and was paralysed. As an experienced psychotherapist, she knew how to deal with transference-love in individual therapy; but now with the baby in the room she was confused. Every act of therapeutic dedication on her part was interpreted and experienced by Mr O as proof of the reality of the romantic sexual relationship between them, as shown by the messages he sent her between sessions; and she felt her ability to maintain her therapeutic stance was severely handicapped. The fact that the baby was present in the room and that there was an actual interaction between the three of them, further blurred the boundary between fantasy and reality. The therapist tried to focus on the father-infant interaction but often felt that Mr O's mind was elsewhere. He declared that Eli was the most important thing in his life, but in the room she felt he didn't pay enough attention to Eli's cues because he only had eyes for her. She began to perceive him as a neglecting father and became worried for the baby. Finally, her distress and frustration reached the point where she suggested that for the benefit of the baby, she should be replaced by another therapist. Following is a detailed description of the one-session supervision that helped her overcome this obstacle and continue the treatment.

The baby at the time was six months old, and the tension between Mr O and the therapist centred on the social worker's recommendation to put Eli in day care. Mr O had begun looking at places, but none seemed good enough for him. The therapist at this point had become adamant about discontinuing her role in the treatment, leaving no room for thought and preventing any possible investigation into the reasons for such an extreme counter-transference. She felt concretely abused and was determined to put an end to it. Therefore, the first step was to help calm her by agreeing to release her from her responsibility for the therapy, so that she could regain her ability to think and process what was going on.

The supervisor agreed to take her place, but she suggested first that they watch the filmed session to try and understand what was going on. The therapist agreed, and they focused on exploring one particular interaction in the session. The supervisor asked the therapist to describe what was happening. Listening to the therapist, the first thing that struck her was that the therapist was giving a description of isolated and unconnected events. Due to her distress, she was apparently unable to see a complete process of interactions between three participants, father, baby, and therapist, which needed to be understood dynamically. The supervisor suggested they look at the segment again, this time with the intention of seeing it as an interactive process. Below is the therapist's second description of the interaction:

- Father complains that the social worker reproached him for delaying the day care solution and allowing other members of the family to care for Eli in an inconsistent way.
- I ask him why he objects so strongly to the day care solution.
- Father's answer is confused and incomprehensible.
- I am silent, thinking he is trying to hide something from me.
- He turns his gaze towards Eli, but seems not to see him because he is so self-absorbed.
- Eli turns his gaze to his father, catches his eye, and they smile at each other.

Now the supervisor noted that the description lacked any affective dimension. They watched the segment a third time, adding the missing affects.

FATHER: 'The social worker told me off for not finding a place for Eli and for letting some family members take care of him.' [His posture, tone of voice and facial expression reflect excitement and embarrassment in the therapist's presence. His words and emotions seem incongruent. There is no affective investment in the baby.]

THERAPIST: 'Why do you object so strongly to day care?' [Angry; sharp dissonance between his warm excitement and her coldness; sense of distance and alienation between father and therapist.]

FATHER: 'Eli . . . day care . . .' [Father tense and frustrated because not understood; therapist feels manipulated, becomes angrier and alert.]

FATHER: (Turns his eyes away from her to baby) [anxious, restless, unfocused.]

ELI: (Perceives his father's gaze; they smile at each other) [Eli is happy; father relaxes.]

After gathering the three dimensions of the interaction-sequential, behavioural and affective-supervisor and therapist can now form a fuller picture of the triadic dynamic. Father feels threatened and reproached when facing the therapist's judgment and criticism of his fatherhood. His need for support remains unrecognised by her because it is defensively disguised by an erotic attitude, which arouses her anger and aversion. In response to her anger his growing anxiety destroys his ability to think and contain his feelings, and his disorganised response is then misinterpreted by her as an attempt to hide something. Now father and therapist face each other defensively, the wall between them rising higher and higher. His uncontained anxiety growing, the disappointed father turns to his son for relief. The therapist misses the intentionality of the father's turning to the baby, thinking he is just turning away from her. The father needs Eli as a calming object, and this is why he cannot let him go to day care. The supervisor suggested that if the therapist could understand that the father needed her to calm him down, his son would be relieved of this burden. The therapist realised that what seemed at first to be a chain of unconnected events was actually an interactive process with three participants, shaped by the dynamics between them.

The therapist suddenly remembered that this interpretation had occurred to her in the session but was somehow forgotten. Later in the session the father told her that Eli was his 'reparation' in life, and she had thought, 'What a burden on little Eli's shoulders!' Then another event from the session came to her mind: Eli's aggressive handling of soft toys. They found the sequence and saw Eli excitedly grab a big, soft stuffed dog, shake it vigorously, then hug and kiss it. The supervisor directed the therapist's attention to the father's reaction. To her surprise, she could now identify his matching affect and the shared feelings of excitement and joy between father and son. It was clearly an experience of affective attunement. The supervisor could now formulate with the therapist a new understanding of the meaning of this scene: it was the appearance of a healthy combination of aggressive and libidinal drives, shared by the two males. The therapist could see their mutual pleasure and joyful connectedness. She realised that a healthy development had taken place as a result of her therapeutic efforts, something she had been unable to see even when she watched the filmed interaction, because of her strong aversion towards the father. She needed the supervisor's eye to recognise and experience herself as an effective therapist. It was a great relief, which enabled her to change her attitude towards Mr O. Encouraged, she decided to continue the treatment. In light of the renewed therapeutic process, the supervisor decided to leave open the question of what in the therapist's inner world had caused her to react so violently to this particular patient. The decision whether such an exploration is necessary within supervision or whether the therapist's personal and intimate material is more suitably dealt with in her own therapy varies among supervisors. In my view, the role of the supervision ends once the therapist regains her ability to think and her therapeutic stance is re-established.

Two insights gained in the supervision had helped to free the therapist from her negative emotional fixation. The first was the recognition of the father's transference love as a sexualisation of his non-sexual need to calm his anxiety. The therapist could now see him as a needy patient and not only an obsessive male suitor. Mr O knew he was bothering her with his insistence but couldn't help himself. Now, with her new understanding, she invited him to an individual session without the protection of Danny's presence. She asked him to stop sending messages, and interpreted his urgent erotic need for her as a transformed defensive expression of his fear of raising his son alone, without a maternal figure. She said she understood his distress but could not accept his behaviour. Now it was clear to both of them-he was a patient and she a therapist. The messages stopped. Although the confrontation was difficult for both parties, their level of anxiety dropped, and so did her aversion. Psychoanalytic therapists are familiar with the theoretical concept of sexualisation, yet the application of this understanding in clinical practice remains complicated, and many therapists can become defensive and confused when they encounter it. Consultation and support from colleagues or analysts are strongly recommended when sexualisation is experienced by the therapist as harassment. In terms of the fatherhood constellation formulated above, Mr O's behaviour would indicate that the anxiety aroused by the necessity to become his son's main caregiver, requiring him to express actual maternal-feminine traits, was related to the destabilising effect of the baby's birth on his male identity; his defensive sexual transference to the therapist would thus serve as a counter-reaction designed to strengthen and support it.

The second insight obtained in the supervision was the realisation of how her negative emotional reaction to the father had narrowed the therapist's ability to 'read the signs' and understand the dynamics unfolding in the room as well as in her mind. Restricted perception is a common defensive mode of adaptation when faced with anxiety. When used by therapists under stress, they may miss not only pathological processes, but also healthy ones set in motion by their interventions. The supervision in this case served as a safe and holding environment that gradually enabled the therapist to expand her perception and thinking until she could regain her therapeutic stance and feel able to see the treatment through to its end, nine months later.

In the first case I described, the therapist's countertransference alone prevented the therapy from proceeding optimally by obscuring from her view what was clearly the father's positive transference and the good working alliance he had formed. This was corrected by her self-analysis and ensuing insight. In the second case, the therapist's negative countertransference came in response to the father's strongly eroticised transference. After the sexualisation had been reinterpreted as a defence against anxiety, caused by the father's neediness and dependency, the therapist could resolve her countertransference, and use it as a source of knowledge about the patient. Only then could she resume her therapeutic stance and respond to the father's underlying need for support and relief from anxiety.

Chapter 10

Working with couples as parents and parents as couples

Louise Emanuel

There is a growing body of research evidence linking sensitive parenting attitudes and secure attachments between parents and their children, with the quality of their couple relationship. The Tavistock Clinic approach to brief psychoanalytically based interventions with parents, infants and young children, increasingly focuses on the importance of the parent-couple relationship, as a key 'port of entry' to understanding underlying family difficulties, with both parents, if available, encouraged to participate. Couple relationship problems impact negatively on parental functioning; young children may be caught up in the disturbing dynamics of polarised parental attitudes, and this may lead to paralysis in the therapist, who feels pulled in two directions by embattled partners; It often emerges that addressing areas of difficulty in the parental relationship can provide relief to children and reduce their symptoms.

Nearly all of the work of the Under Fives Service is done in the presence of one or both parents, either with the child or on their own. Often the focus is on helping the parents to gain the insight and strength to function together as a benign parental couple, despite sometimes conscious or unconscious attempts by the child to split the couple. In other cases, work may centre on helping a 'single' parent understand her child's need for her to exercise both paternal and maternal functions: to maintain in her mind, and to cultivate in the child's mind, the notion of a well-functioning parental couple. Underlying this approach to work with parents and children is the idea that each parent embodies within him/herself both a paternal and a maternal function, a combined internal parental couple. This links with Bion's (1962) concept of container/contained. Bion's concept of a 'container' incorporates both the maternal receptive and the paternal 'structuring, penetrative' role – a new thought, a transformation of what is received. Thus it is essential for the development of a capacity to think symbolically that a child internalises a parental object with both paternal and maternal functions.

The 'paternal function' is characterised by benign but firm boundary and limit setting, a capacity for 'penetrative' insight (new ideas and initiatives) and the 'maternal function' is characterised by tender receptivity to a child's communications of both pleasure and distress. The combination of these qualities of both firmness and receptivity provides a containing framework within which children in both single and two parent families are able to flourish.

These functions can often become polarised in poorly functioning parent couples where one parent of either gender may embody an extreme (parodied) version of a 'paternal function' (i.e. be excessively punitive and harsh, restrictive rather than limit-setting) or of a 'maternal function' (i.e. be excessively indulgent and permissive, lacking any limit-setting capacity). Parents of both genders can embody either function. This may be linked to the ways in which each parent has (unconsciously or consciously) chosen to respond to their own parental background, if there has been a history of abuse, either identifying with a harsh punitive paternal figure or reacting against it, resulting in a difficulty in setting firm limits. Serious couple/marital difficulties often underlie the parenting problems and can prove intractable.

Underlying this approach to work with parents and children is the idea that each parent embodies within him/herself both a paternal and a maternal function, a combined internal parental couple. I will give a brief vignette of the kind of drama where the extreme splits between the parents are brought into dramatic relief, for work within family and parent sessions.

Two-year-old Gareth was referred for severe tantrums, head-banging and concerns because of speech delay. I was alerted to the extreme split between these parents in the waiting room, as they were seated so far apart I couldn't identify them as a couple. Gareth ran out and set off on his own in the opposite direction. Father grabbed him forcibly and brought him to the room. In the room Gareth sat next to father on the couch, but mother showed him to the little chair at the table. It felt as if they were pulling in opposite directions from the start. Gareth was unsettled and restless, and did not ask once for help to lift toys or take lids off pens. He struck me as prematurely self-sufficient, avoiding interaction with any of us. Mother spoke loudly and constantly, father sat surly and quiet, just repeating 'head-banging' when I asked about his concerns.

It became apparent that their styles of discipline were extremely different. Father appeared to be much stricter, and his voice exuded a quiet controlled threat of violence – 'I just raise my finger and he listens'; Mother seemed much 'softer' on Gareth, allowed him to rummage in her bag and tip its entire contents onto the floor of my room. She told me she 'doesn't believe in routine, Gareth will have routines for the rest of his life', so he had no fixed bed time and fell asleep on the sofa.

Gareth demonstrated a tantrum when I stopped him using my computer, banging his head violently against mother's legs and on the floor, becoming very distressed. To comfort him mother produced a half empty tube of 'cream', which he held and squeezed, like a soft comforting breast. Mother told me he took it to bed and woke up grasping for it; he loved soft fabrics and comforters and took them everywhere.

He made baby sounds in public and hardly spoke. Father was concerned about Gareth wearing mother's shoes and handbags around the house. I said it was unlikely to be a gender identity issue but rather Gareth's way of 'becoming' mummy, having total access to her. The split between the self-sufficient boy and the tiny baby, Gareth paralleled the split between the parents.

As well as attending nursery Gareth was being cared for by both set of grandparents, mother, and father all in shifts, each one imposing their own very different sets of expectations on him. I suspected that he was being driven 'crazy' with worry about how he had to behave at any one time, the stress of adapting from one kind of care to another being too great for him to cope with. He was becoming hyper-vigilant, and 'disorganised' in his behaviour, unable to predict from hour to hour what behaviour was expected of him. I thought his frustration and anxiety might be calmed by his parents getting together to think about how they could unite in their approach to his care. In subsequent meetings mother and father found it difficult to accept the ways in which each disciplined Gareth. This was clearly linked to their own troubled histories of abuse and abandonment – each had chosen a different response, with mother determined not to do the same, feeling that any separation or boundary would be cruel (her own history had been of sudden loss), and father by identifying with the rather menacing figures in his early life.

The parents' own internal difficulties manifested themselves in this *external drama* – the dysfunctional polarised parenting, where the extreme lack of boundaries in mother, which allowed him to 'merge' totally with her and where language would be perceived to be unnecessary, and the over-punitive father, resulted in dysfunctional parenting which was impacting negatively on Gareth's life. Over time things shifted slightly, with father becoming a little more receptive towards Gareth and mother becoming a little more boundaried with him. Gareth's head banging diminished although it was clear that his problems and the family's were complex, and more help would be required.

In his paper, P. Barrows (2004), having discussed the 'ghosts' that haunt the nursery (Fraiberg, 1987), argues that work with the parent/couple on the 'intimacy of the marital relationship' is an important and valid part of work with families with children under five, 'given the importance of the nature of the couple's relationship for the infant's psychological development'. He argues that, having established the existence of 'unprocessed trauma in the parent's background', work with the parental couple needs to take place in the 'here and now' because 'what matters from the infant's point of view is not so much *whose* ghost it is, father's or mother's, but the nature of the interaction that then ensues between the parents' (Barrows, 2004).

Oedipal issues and the parental couple

I would like to address the feelings of exclusion and separateness commonly experienced by the young child, and remaining a feature of adolescents and some adults (see my adult patient) as he moves away from the exclusive relationship with his primary carer, usually mother, and towards triangular relationship, most notably with father, but also with siblings, and often a new baby. I will describe therapeutic work with a family struggling with conflicts, anxieties and defences associated with the triangular constellation of mother, father and child – the Oedipal situation. Not only does the child begin to perceive his parents as a couple from whose relationship he can be excluded; he also recognises, in the words of Hanna Segal, that

> the nature of the link between the parents is different in kind from the relation of the child to the parents and at the moment unavailable to him . . . It is not only that they exchange genital gratifications, but also the fact that the parental intercourse leads to the creation of a new baby.
>
> (Segal, 1989)

This realisation of parental sexuality and partnership, as well as his growing awareness of difference between adults and children, will inevitably generate very strong feelings of loss, envy and jealousy. Rivalry with one parent for the attention of the other is a common consequence of such recognition. However, it may also encourage him to find comfort in other relationships and activities, most significantly with his father.

Working through these ordinary but painful anxieties and conflicts is facilitated by the presence of a securely based internal parental couple in the child's mind. The absence of a 'united' parental couple can make it more complicated for the child to establish an Oedipal triangle. Parents' own unresolved Oedipal conflicts could lead them to over-identify with their child, thus discouraging separation and growth. The birth of a new baby can stir up a sense of displacement in the child, and this in turn might make parents feel guilty and reluctant to set ordinary boundaries. There is always the child's own personality and unique way of perceiving and interpreting parental and sibling behaviour to be taken into account, too.

The resolution of the Oedipal situation through relinquishing the sole possession of mother and the acceptance of the parents' relationship with each other creates what Ronald Britton calls 'a triangular space'.

Oedipal rivalry

This case illustrates a common family problem: a two-year-old who feels pushed out of place after the birth of a sibling. In this case the little girl turned to her father for comfort, as little girls often do; but in her mind this took on unusual proportions, as in her imagination she had rearranged the family into a new set of couples: herself and father on one side and mother and baby brother on the other. This was her way of denying the fact of her parents' intimate couple relationship.

Mrs A contacted the local child guidance service asking for help with her two-and-a-half-year-old daughter, Maria, due to her waking up frequently at night and demanding mother's sole attention during the day, unable to play on her own. The family was under strain at the time of referral, with maternal grandmother suffering from cancer. In addition the family's home was undergoing some renovation and was in chaos.

Although the whole family was invited for the first meeting mother chose to come on her own.

Mrs A became very tearful as she spoke about the burden she was carrying: the care of her two children, Maria and Daniel (11 months old) as well as her own parents, particularly now that her mother was very ill. She said that both she and her husband were bewildered by the change in Maria. She used to be a wonderful baby before her brother was born and in the last few months has become so demanding and clingy, day and night, that both parents were on verge of collapse. The baby, however, appeared very calm and contented and slept through the night.

Mrs A herself was calmer by the end of the meeting and was able to link Maria's difficulties to the strained situation at home, while she was already having to struggle with the arrival of her new baby brother. We spoke about Mrs A's fear of losing her own mother and the way both mother and daughter shared the same fears of abandonment.

The princess

A more convenient, after-work time and mother's sense of relief after the first meeting seemed to enable the whole family to attend the second session. Mother's initial description of her older daughter as anxious and sensitive did not prepare me for the picture I was presented with. Maria appeared as a very self-assured, domineering 'princess', whose long hair fell elegantly over her face like a veil, also keeping her eyes quite hidden. Her presence in the room as a central figure was unquestionable, while her younger brother seemed to be rather inconspicuous. Mr A was quiet to begin with but did not come across as suspicious of this kind of work in the way that his wife had anticipated.

Maria went straight to the table where a few drawing materials were laid out and she stayed standing by the table, presumably to keep her height (or highness!) at all times. There was also a sense of her not really needing anything that was on offer here, as if she was just passing by or on her way to somewhere more interesting. She started drawing offhandedly many circles on one sheet of paper followed by another and another. She then distributed them to all people present in a dramatic, teacher-like manner. Mother explained that Maria was presently learning about triangles, squares and circles, 'but circles are her favourite' (I thought of her need to be in the centre, within a circle, as in a bubble/couple rather than within a triangle or square, shapes that are associated with more than two. A triangle, with its apex and sharp corners, could be associated with feelings of exclusion and loneliness highlighted by the sharpness of the edges, in contrast to the soft never-ending shape of a circle.) On completing this activity she found herself having nothing to do (as if having to face being a child in the corner) and the tension in the room started rising as she began to grab things from her brother, who faintly protested. When parents made a mild comment about this, Maria immediately veered towards mother's bag full of 'bribes', (sweets), which mother said she takes 'just in case'.

Maria, moved swiftly to sit on her father's lap, spreading herself all over him, and proceeding to command him to get her this or that. Father did not challenge her, yet I could not help but notice how determined she was in avoiding eye contact with me. I thought that she probably perceived me as a threat to the status quo.

I heard from mother that in the night she wakes up and comes to her parents' bedroom. Mother does not like her getting into their bed so father usually takes her back to her own bed and stays with her until she falls asleep. (I thought that although the parents were clear in keeping their bed out of bounds, Maria did manage to get her father out of the matrimonial bed and have him all to herself. Her waking up several times at night could be triggered by her fear that he would slip back to mother.) During the day however she follows mother everywhere and demands her exclusive attention. (Out of guilt for taking her husband away from her? Or a way of being mother's shadow, as if by sticking close to mother she can instantly 'become' mother, and avoid having to know about being a little girl.)

I asked the parents whether they thought Maria might be checking on them at night, as she seemed to have a very strong need to be right in the middle so as not to feel excluded. Both parents were amused by this and mother became more animated and said simply: 'Oh yes, Maria is married to her father'. I said that she seemed therefore to be in competition with mother who is already married to her husband. Here Maria became very upset and strongly protested: '*My* daddy! Mummy is Daniel's mummy and Daddy is *mine*'. Mother said that sometimes she teases Maria by saying, 'He is *my* husband' and Maria protests back: 'No, he is *my* daddy'.

As we continued to talk about this Maria asked mother for her ring (her wedding ring was the only one on her finger) and mother let her have it. In gratitude Maria offered her kindly her own cheap plastic one. I was reminded of the circles and Maria's dislike of triangles and squares while circles may be evocative of a couple enclosed with no corners to bump against. (The wedding ring circle as a symbol of the relationship between mother and father.)

This prompted a lively conversation as the parents began to show more interest in understanding aspects of their daughter's behaviour. They were able to recognise that Maria's night-time waking and day-time clinging to mother during father's absence at work illustrated her need to keep an eye on her parents, partly to make sure that they do not produce any more babies, as it were, but also to protect herself against feeling abandoned (it is likely that her increased hostility and intrusiveness would have brought greater fear of retaliation and abandonment).

There was also a fear of being left with nothing, particularly as Maria would perceive her baby brother as snatching her own place with mother. They could also see her following mother's footsteps as not only literally clinging or gluing herself to her but as also wishing to *be* her, in order not to be faced with the painful reality of the difference between her and her mother, who after all produced lovely babies. The parents were both relieved and keen to proceed with the work.

Although I could see that the current situation at home may have exacerbated Maria's need to keep a vigilant eye on her parents I was not yet clear what made it difficult for these parents to manage her demands and bear her feelings. I wondered whether some of these difficulties were already experienced prior to the arrival of the new baby but were intensified by his birth. Perhaps Maria was a particularly demanding, envious baby who had found it especially difficult to bear the position of needing mother and perceiving her as the holder of all good things. Certainly both parents seemed to find it very difficult to challenge her in an ordinary way: they were almost too empathetic towards Maria, understanding her discomfort and frustration and wishing only to take those feelings away. Linking to their own childhood, it looked as if they were both very identified with her vulnerable feelings and were therefore less able to take a parental stance of setting boundaries in a clear albeit friendly manner, perhaps for fear of hurting her and possibly becoming unpopular in Maria's eyes. This in turn fed into her omnipotence and the picture of being at one with her parents. Their helplessness therefore made her feel all too powerful, thus controlling her own vulnerable part in a rather grotesque way. In the third and subsequent meetings, parents reported improvements, in Maria's sleep and behaviour during the day, and further work led to increased resolution of the problem, and a stronger, more united parental couple.

There is no time to develop these themes further, but it is helpful to recognise that offering a containing space in which the emotional needs of fathers and the parental couple can be met, and which may involve alternating family meetings with separate parent sessions, is important. Psychoanalyst Bion's concept of 'container/contained', and Britton's concept of the therapist who can provide a 'third position', on the various points of view within the family, are valuable theoretical frameworks.

Chapter 11

Can the difficulties of carrying out the paternal function for a toddler be identified from the earliest months of a baby's life?

Marie-Christine Laznik

Introduction: what is the paternal function?

It is not easy to speak about the paternal function in clinical work with babies. For Lacan, the key aspect of the role of the real father, the mother's partner, consists in separating, at a certain moment, the mother from her child and the child from his mother, in order to introduce the child into the register of symbolic exchange, and thus allow him to himself become a father one day. In this text, I will focus on the male child, because, one, the two clinical examples I discuss concern boys and, two, the question of the dissolution of the Oedipus complex, in which the father plays a crucial role, is simpler.

However, this role is not the same as that performed by a dad for a newborn, who primarily needs help reducing the internal and external excitations, and who can only start noticing the words and gaze of the helpful Other, Freud's *Nebenmench* (Freud, 1950 [1895], p. 317), once this tension has been reduced. The founding scene of the baby's narcissism, so aptly represented in the Nativity scene, where everyone congregates around His Majesty the Baby, can only take place if the baby does not suffer. The baby's well-being is the primordial task of the mother and the dad helps her as best as he can. Yet this assistance does not constitute the paternal function properly speaking. In the Nativity scene, Joseph's often puzzled expression conveys his confusion and perplexity. Sharing in the maternal care, as it is often the case today, does not make one more of a father. A good dad, yes – but not a father. Still, the question of the possibility of there later being a real father for the child is implicitly present from the very beginning.

Already for Freud, the question of '*What is a father?*' remained enigmatic. In today's society, where the struggle for gender equality has often led to a confusion between the roles of the father and the mother, the question becomes even more obscure.

It is interesting to listen to two young parents speaking about this question while their baby is sleeping. However, to understand the relevance of their conversation as well as the pertinence (or lack thereof) of the analyst's interventions, we must first look at the clinical case of a slightly older child, a two-year-old. Patrick teaches us a valuable lesson about the importance of the function of the real father, a lesson I consider to be even richer than the one transmitted by Little Hans to Freud and Lacan. It was Patrick who showed me that Lacan's commentary on the case of Little Hans remains just as relevant today.

Part I: Patrick, or the dangers of a father's refusal to play his role

Patrick is two years old when his mother gets in touch with our team at the Centre Alfred Binet in Paris. She asks for an appointment because, as she says, her son has been 'violent towards his parents'.

When I meet them, the mother relays the complaints received from the nursery: 'Patrick fights not just with other children, hitting and biting them, but also with the adults, whom he kicks, which the nursery absolutely cannot tolerate. This is an emergency.'

I make a place for him at a little table and offer him different toys. From the outset, Patrick shows a striking imaginative capacity, even though the game he plays will long remain utterly repetitive.

While his mother is speaking to me about him, about his birth and the first months of his life, Patrick creates a puzzling scenario. I should say that I only realised how crucial this scenario was thanks to his determination in showing me its different versions.

Among the boxes of toys, Patrick chooses a family of animals and four pieces of fence. A daddy horse, a mummy horse and a baby horse. He names them accordingly. A fight breaks out between Daddy-horse and Baby-horse, in which the baby, despite its smaller size, seems to win and kicks the dad out of the house. Daddy-horse falls on the ground and the little one stays alone with his mother.

A few minutes later, Patrick goes through another box, looking for the giant monster he has previously seen there. 'Monster' is his own word. For this role, he chooses a prehistoric animal that is much bigger than the other animals in the box. We also have a lion and a tiger of the same size as the adult horse, but Patrick instead chooses this giant 'monster'.

On its arrival, the monster starts breaking the walls of the house, represented by the fence, which falls to the floor. It then attacks the mother, who does not defend herself: it is true that she's much smaller than the monster. Then the baby is annihilated and falls off the table, as if falling into the void.

Patrick soon reproduces the scenario with different characters. The same scene takes place, this time with the cow family and the bull. Patrick is very attentive to the genitals as they are represented in these figures. It is indeed the bull, with his male attributes, whom he names 'Daddy', while the cow occupies the place of the mother. Like in the horse family, he chooses a little calf to play the baby. He creates a new house with the pieces of fence, where he places the three characters. Soon the calf starts attacking the father, who is much bigger – the animals are appropriately differentiated in size – and again wins the battle. The father is expelled from the house and falls into the hole.

Seeing my surprise, the mother confirms that her husband refuses to exert any kind of authority over their son, blaming the little time he has with him, which he prefers to spend playing with him. She complains that she alone has to bear the dimension of severity required to discipline her son.

Next in the game there is a moment of tranquillity between the calf and the mother cow, which is soon disturbed by the arrival of the monster. While the family characters change, the monster is always the same large prehistoric animal, huge compared to the rest of the characters. The monster arrives, destroys the house, attacks the mother who still cannot defend herself – she is indeed a lot smaller – and crushes the baby, who finds himself in the hole. In the two weekly sessions before the summer holidays, I will see this scenario played out numerous times.

Before looking at the rest of the treatment, let us try and see what this scene can teach us. It seems reasonable to argue that what we see is the little boy's entrance into the Oedipus complex, where the inaugural scene shows us the rivalry between father and son, the latter trying to eliminate his rival in order to preserve the exclusive enjoyment of the mother. Patrick does not deny the difference in size between the father and the son, but he indicates that the father is very weak, and his tiny son can easily eliminate him. The desire of this two-year-old follows the logic of Freud's argument about little Hans, which he pronounces during their first meeting: 'Long before he was in the world ... I had known that a little Hans would come who would be so fond of his mother that he would be bound to feel afraid of his father because of it' (Freud, 1909b, p. 41). Freud makes this interpretation after he has listened to Hans talking about the horse and making him associate on the similarity between the horse and his father.

Let's not forget that Hans' father is rather startled by this, because he is extremely gentle with his son and does all he can for Hans not to feel any hostility towards him. He cannot comprehend how the child could possibly be afraid of him. Patrick's mother describes a father who resembles that of Freud's little patient. In both cases, there seems to be a failure of the paternal function.

Patrick has not yet formed a phobia and we cannot know whether he will do so at a later time. At the moment, he is less than half of Hans' age and the latter did not previously show any aggressive or violent behaviour towards adults. It is true that their backgrounds are very different. Hans had an entire court around him, constantly at his disposal, while Patrick has to deal with the harsh collective life of the nursery. However, Patrick is also fond of his giant destructive animal. He does not seem scared of it; rather he seems waiting for it to appear, as if it played a crucial role – but what role? Following Freud's direction, we could notice that its arrival puts an end to the mother-child relationship, albeit in a radical way: by destroying everything.

In his essay 'Inhibitions, Symptoms and Anxiety', Freud argues, regarding Hans' fear of horses, that the phobic animal is always a paternal substitute (Freud, 1926a, p. 103). In the same year, in 'The Question of Lay Analysis', he again states this clearly: the animal is 'a disguise of the father' (Freud, 1926b, p. 210). Yet in his case, the child does experience anxiety.

The question of anxiety and its absence is discussed in *Totem and Taboo*, specifically in the chapter entitled 'The Return of Totemism in Childhood' (Freud, 1913, p. 99). Freud mentions the clinical account by Dr Wulff, of a child who loved the dogs that could bite him so much that he would openly declare his love to them (p. 127). Freud is himself somewhat puzzled by this absence of anxiety, but he maintains that these observations justify us 'in substituting the father for the totem animal' (p. 130). The absence of anxiety, as well as the love for the biting animal, would suggest that faced with the danger of maternal engulfment, for which it is a metaphoric substitution, the monster is a very fortunate discovery. This line of argument remains quite Freudian.

In his paper on 'Aggressiveness in Psychoanalysis' (Lacan, 2005), Lacan's argument is based on criminological data; he says that he is struck by the force commanding certain delinquents, who act as if they were *fulfilling an order*. Could this possibility help us understand Patrick's aggressive behaviour at the nursery? If so, we might be concerned that Patrick's future harbours something else than a phobia. We will of course never know, because the analytic encounter has changed the course of events.

Continuation of the clinical material

The family returns after the summer holidays, in September. With extreme rigour, Patrick again repeats the two previously described scenarios.

In November, I finally meet the father, who brings his son while the mother is away. The father says he feels overwhelmed by the son's aggressiveness at the nursery, but he does not complain of his behaviour at home. He even says that he loves playing with Patrick and lets him win whenever they play at a battle. He thinks that pretending to lose to his little son in order to make him feel really strong is great fun. And so, whenever they physically play-fight, he lets him win. He tells me about all this with great amusement. He repeats what his wife has already told me: that he is often away for work and wants to take advantage of his time with Patrick, wants to enjoy it rather than spend it disciplining him: 'I'd like him to think of me as his friend, rather than his father.' I try to explain to the father that his position makes his son an orphan of his father, and thus exposed to anxiety. I can see that the father has no idea what I am talking about – it is Patrick who helps make things clearer, who, so to say, lays the cards on the table.

During this long discussion with the father, Patrick goes to look for his toys and recreates his habitual scenario on the little table.

While Patrick's father is watching, puzzled, the baby animal again wins over its father and is left alone with the mother; soon the monster arrives and destroys everything, killing both mother and baby. During the first enactment, I feel that the father still cannot quite believe what he is looking at, namely the havoc wreaked on a child by the absence of a strong father worthy of his name.

However, the repetition of the same scene with different animals, right in front of the father's nose, makes him think that the giant beast might perhaps represent the external dangers threatening his son. Slowly, he comes to admit that the child might indeed feel in danger, alone and helpless against the other children at the nursery who, no doubt, are not always very nice to him. The father has more difficulty admitting that the monster could also be an emanation of the son's fantasy life.

During this time, Patrick continues replaying the scene with a family of elephants. Despite the daddy's large size, the little elephant easily beats him. The arrival of the monster, still the same, ends in total destruction. As I comment on the scene and especially the baby's terrible annihilation by the monster, the father suddenly remembers the nightmares disturbing his son's sleep.

As I have done with the mother, I again praise the son's dramatic abilities and the psychoanalytic precision of his representations. I have to say that throughout my career as an analyst, which spans over forty years, I had never before encountered such a rigorous staging, by a child, of the question of the failure of the paternal function. In order to lighten the mood, I ask the father if he might not have actually read some psychoanalytic texts to his son.

Relaxing slightly, the father says no, but that he can see what it is his son is trying to show. He mentions a 1980s film, *Airplane!* (in French aptly renamed *Is There a Pilot on Board?*). In the story, the terrified passengers realise that the plane they are travelling on might not actually be under anyone's control.

Two weeks later, I ask both parents to come see me. The mother complains of the fact that the father refuses to discipline their son, leaving this unpleasant role to her. The father says he has thought about the scene his son showed him, but he finds the idea of disciplining him repulsive.

I hear myself say:

> I am simply asking you to give the little ship's boy the feeling that there is a captain on board and that if he obeys him, all dangers will be avoided. I am not asking you to play the sergeant and scream at him.

The father grows pale and says:

> Madame, my father is an army sergeant. I've spent my childhood in military barracks because of his relocations. I've always hated the fact that he would only scream at home. I swore to myself that when I have a child, I will do the exact opposite: I will be my son's friend.

The three of us took some time to absorb what has just been revealed. We then spoke about the repetitive scenarios staged by the boy many times before the mother and father, using different animals. I again speak about the son's accurate representation of the weak father and the unavoidable catastrophe that follows. I tell them it is completely in line with psychoanalytic theory and we joke that, like Obelix, baby Patrick must have fallen into a psychoanalytic cauldron, in order to be so knowledgeable at such an early age.

Patrick's case is a wonderful example of what Lacan tried to articulate regarding the little boy's Oedipal complex. He writes:

> He is, as the Freudian dialectic describes him, a little criminal. It is via this imaginary crime that he enters the order of the law. But he cannot enter it unless he has had, at least for a moment, a real partner facing him.
> (Lacan, 1998a, pp. 209–10)

Lacan's argument concerns little Hans, but Patrick is an even better example.

The father says that he has never thought that by playing the role of a friend, he would leave his son feeling helpless against the dangers of life. He speaks about his hostility aimed at, if not his own father, then the latter's child-rearing methods. In order not the throw out the baby with the bathwater, he says he will try to radically change his position. Using the monster scenario, I talk to them about a child's inner psychic life, its currents and terrifying monsters.

To my great surprise, as soon as the father changes his position and assumes his role as a real father, Patrick makes swift progress. Already before the Christmas holidays, the scenario has changed: the family is still there, but now the daddy brings the boy to school every morning. The little elephant – because this is now the animal family Patrick prefers – happily follows his father, the big elephant.

Patrick is now three years old and the school no longer has any complaints. The parents have a lot of fun with him. The father holds his place as a real father; the mother seems very relieved. I never see the scene with the destroying monster again. In the stories he now stages, the father plays rather a protective role. As if the father's reversal allowed the little boy to rally under his banner – a kind of resolution, albeit a rather early one, of the Oedipus complex. The symptoms the parents complained about have disappeared. We decide to end the treatment, which lasted for fourteen sessions.

Theoretical considerations

How do we account for this rather spectacular improvement, as soon as the real father enters the scene? In order to do so, we must first look at the child's symptoms in the light of their disappearance.

We see that the monster prevented the little boy from taking the kind of megalomaniac position we see in our work with psychotic children, where the child wins at everything, regardless of common sense.

Here, should we wish to use Freudian terms, castration is not possible. The monster destroys everything – there is no negotiation. What then could be its function?

The monster prevents the boy from fantasising about the danger of the mother reincorporating her own product – himself. The devouring figure is not the mother, who is instead pictured as just as fragile as himself and who is destroyed together with the house.

The scene thus spares the maternal imago and the tender bond with the mother, by projecting all her dangerous and devouring aspects onto the figure of the monster, external to the family. Let's not forget that before coming here and finding an extremely attentive audience in the person of the analyst, Patrick was violent with his mother and the – mostly female – staff at the nursery. The father saw his son's aggressiveness against himself as a game, in which he enjoyed letting the boy win.

With regards to the monster, I also thought about the more intrapsychic dimension of the subject, the locus of the sadistic dimension of his drives, even though in this case the archaic superego remained unconnected to symbolic castration. I was very surprised at the quasi-immediate subjective transformation of not just the child's behaviour towards others, but also of the scene staged by him.

The reason why the child gave up so easily on the aspects of the scene that seemed to properly engage the drives, such as the aggressive behaviour towards others, both big and small, was because the benefit of this renunciation was bigger than the fear of annihilation provoked by the non-mediated fantasmatic maternal figure. We can only recognise this as the pacifying dimension of the Oedipal resolution for a non-psychotic boy. As we have seen, it required the intervention of a real father, certainly loving, but now also taking his position as the ship's captain – to the ship's boy's greatest relief.

Indeed, what is a real father? The function comprises several registers. As Lacan argued, for the child not to feel at risk of being engulfed by the mother, the function of the father must be recognised, so that he can deprive her of her child, while showing her his love (Lacan, 2017, p. 153). This privation constitutes the first denting in the maternal 'other'. When this first register of the paternal function is inactive, the monster can help 'imaginarise' the necessary dent in the primordial maternal 'other'.

It seems that in this first stage, things worked out for Patrick: the place of the third existed, even though his father did not embody it. The mother in a sense indicated to her son that there was indeed a phallus beyond himself. However, the psyche of little boys needs to find a figure to embody the father in reality: this is the real father. His role is to deprive the baby of his mother and vice versa – all the better if he also has a place in the mother's bed. In this case, the little subject can submit to the father, who is now considered as ideal.

Part II: The complexity of the paternal function in the work with infants

In our everyday work with children who begin to show behavioural problems at around two or three years of age, I am most often faced with mothers who wish to rule the family home. It seems that in many of these cases, the psyche of little boys does not react very well to such arrangement. As if their unconscious was not 'politically correct'. When the law is not held by a third agent, it is not experienced by the child as a law, but as abuse coming from a tyrant with whom they are locked in a combat. They will then rebel against any form of law imposed in their social environment: at home, at the nursery or maternity school.

In these cases, we nearly always see the same scenario: a father who cannot perform his role as a father. With one difference: in many of the cases, the mothers do not see why the law of the mother could not be just as effective in raising a little boy. This seems consistent with today's social discourse on gender equality. There is a relatively widespread confusion between 'gender equality' and 'equality of the mother and the father'.[1] The fact that little Patrick reacted to the treatment so quickly was because his mother did not stand in the way of the paternal function. It was her husband who had rejected this function, due to his refusal to identify with his father.

After a futile conflict, the father often lets the mother do as she pleases, giving up on his own role. In the transference work with mothers, I have most often been able to help them give up on their role as the boss, as the enunciator of the law, even if it is only for a few days, and let the father do his job instead. Because their little boy then usually makes spectacular symptomatic progress, they often come back to ask me to help them maintain this rather theatrical position of letting the father be 'in charge'. However, in all of these cases, the work with the mother turned out to be essential, which was not the case for Patrick's mother.

Against the background of this clinical experience, it is interesting to listen to the dialogue of the parents of a five-month-old baby, which again brought up many of the same issues articulated by the parents I have described. It suggests that the fathers' later difficulties in taking up their role are rooted in a much earlier period, when the child is still a small baby.

This dialogue was recorded as part of a treatment of a baby considered at 'high risk of autism', whose three-year-old brother had previously been diagnosed with an autistic spectrum disorder according to the DSM-5 criteria. The older brother had been treated not only by a psychoanalyst but by a multidisciplinary team and the treatment had proven beneficial; the parents have a very positive transference to me, as I was the person to have referred them to the relevant specialists. When Ulysse, the younger brother, was born, I promised the parents that I would assess the baby; in the case of a risk, we would start treatment immediately. And in fact, baby Ulysse initially presented as very withdrawn.

What follows is a transcription of a session at a time when the baby is already doing much better: it is an interesting session, because it highlights the question of the paternal function.

As part of our research on babies considered at high risk of autism and with the parents' consent, these sessions are filmed. I should explain that the following dialogue is not at all related to the risk of autism.

These are very fine parents, very alert, and the mother, who trusts me, speaks openly about her feelings. Her words reflect the values of our society, in which the 'decline of the *nom du père*' has made room for fantasies of 'omniscience' quite common among mothers.

During this session, Ulysse is asleep: this has not happened before. I thus decide to have a chat with the parents. I tell them that the baby's osteopath, to whom I had sent them, rightly scolded me for not referring the baby to her earlier than at four-and-a-half months. She thought this was a serious problem, because the baby, who had been born with the umbilical cord wrapped around his neck, should have come earlier. Already in the first session, when he was one-and-a-half months old, I saw that the baby was in great physical discomfort; I know that the babies considered at 'high risk of autism' nearly always show problems of bodily organisation. I had trusted the movement therapist[2] to whom I had initially sent the baby, but she did not take the umbilical cord into consideration. We had both been wrong, I tell the parents.

The reason why I mention this staging of the psychoanalyst's 'mistake' is that it had certainly allowed the following discussion to unfold. The fact that the analyst presented herself as having made a mistake made it possible for the mother to then question herself as well. Here is the scene as it was recorded:

We are all admiring the beautiful sleeping baby.

LAZNIK TO THE FATHER: He's such a darling, I wonder how you can leave for work and stop looking at him.

FATHER: It's true, it's really hard.

MOTHER: We're the mummy hen and daddy chicken.

LAZNIK: Daddy-rooster, excuse me! A chicken is the hen's child! That's not on!

The father bursts out laughing.

LAZNIK: Let's put the baby back into his bed, because it's Daddy-rooster! It means a lot, to be the head of the hen house!

In fact, since his birth, Ulysse has been sleeping in the parents' bed, pressed against his mother, and my various interventions in this matter have had zero effect. When he would be put back in his cot, he would stay asleep for about forty minutes maximum, and so every night it would continue.

MOTHER: I sometimes feel like it's me, the head of the hen house.

LAZNIK: Well then, there's something to work on, because it has to be the father who has to *cock-a-doodle-doo* at home. He will have to, he's got two sons.

MOTHER: I don't know, but it's me who takes the books from Alexandre [the son aged three] when it's bedtime, it's me who says "no" all the time. [Turning to the father:] You never say 'no'!

LAZNIK: Perhaps it doesn't bother him that Alexandre's reading a bit late in the evening.

MOTHER: If you leave him the book it can go on until really late. So, I think, as his mum, that he will be tired.

LAZNIK: You don't ask Daddy what he thinks, before you intervene? What does Mr Daddy think?

THE FATHER, PREVIOUSLY VERY QUIET, SAYS: Is that a question?

LAZNIK: Yes.

FATHER: I think we should leave him be, because he'll fall asleep naturally. I used to like reading in my bedroom in the evening and my parents didn't know anything.

LAZNIK: That must have been later, no?

MOTHER: At some point, should a parent decide what's good for their child? Yes!

LAZNIK COMMENTS: Mum doesn't leave much space here; the answer comes before Dad's been able to give his opinion.

The father says he is worried about what we are going to think of his answer, but he agrees to go for it anyway.

FATHER: I am for nearly absolute freedom.

MOTHER: No! Absolute freedom destroys freedom!

FATHER, SLIGHTLY ANGRY: But I did not say that!

MOTHER: You did, it comes down to the same thing!

THE FATHER GIVES UP: OK.

MOTHER: My father was just like you.

LAZNIK, TRYING TO LIGHTEN THE SITUATION: And now we know why Mum chose Dad!

Both parents laugh and the atmosphere becomes slightly more relaxed.

LAZNIK (SPEAKING TO BOTH PARENTS): This is taking us away from our immediate concerns, but these are interesting questions. Between the toxic situation of your little boy being so tired for a while and the fact that it's Mummy who makes the law at home, it's clear: the first is a less serious problem than the second.

MOTHER: I have no problem saying no to my son, because I am more and more able to trust my own judgment.

LAZNIK: Mummy and her 'judgment'! You'll need to learn to let go. We mothers have all had the same thought: We know what's best. Myself, I hold on to my chair and say: Perhaps I'm right, but it will be the way father says!

Laznik mimes the scene in which she is holding onto her chair and the mother starts laughing.

THE FATHER LOOKS AMUSED: The more I'm getting to know you, Mrs Laznik, the more I like you! *He laughs.*

LAZNIK: In order for little boys to grow up, you must overcome this absolute conviction that we, the good mothers, all share: that we know what is best for our child.

The mother laughs The fact that the psychoanalyst includes herself in the difficulty that mothers have in giving up their omnipotence eliminates the superegoic charge of her words. It allows the mother to identify with the analyst. We also have to keep in mind that this mother has been deeply wounded by the illness of her eldest son and learning how to trust her intuition again has been a very important step for her.

LAZNIK: We mothers must learn how to bite our tongues.

All this conversation happens in a warm and relaxed atmosphere, which is what makes it possible.

THE MOTHER THEN SPEAKS ABOUT THE ADVENTURE ON A VENICE GONDOLA: But I have a husband who banged his head against a bridge in Venice, because he was not paying attention. *Laznik points out to her that in the coming years she might also bang her head against something, yet this does not disqualify her as a parent.*

LAZNIK: You know, with super-protective mothers, who think that the father is a chicken in their hen house, you know where that leads? It leads to behaviour problems in little boys, at the maternity school. So, we have to learn that even though we think we are right, we have to let the father do things his way.

THE FATHER LAUGHS. HIS WIFE SAYS TO HIM, IN AN AMUSED TONE: Do you realise this is going to kill me?

LAZNIK: But the results are extraordinary, especially for the little boys.

The mother then asks me if the father might not do something that would put the child's safety at risk.

LAZNIK: You know how much I respect you, enough to think that the man you have chosen to be the father of your children is neither stupid nor crazy.

MOTHER: It's paradoxical, sometimes I have a tendency to think he is. He himself tells me: 'But do you think I'm stupid?'

LAZNIK: You don't have enough confidence in yourself, because I am sure you have chosen a very good man.

MOTHER: The worst thing is that I am convinced of it.

LAZNIK: If you don't provoke him, his children will not get ill. He loves his children.

MOTHER: Of course he loves them. I tell everyone that he's a wonderful father.

LAZNIK: With such a wonderful father, one can feel a bit crushed. For us mothers who know-it-all, it's difficult! *Everyone laughs.*

MOTHER: So what are we going to do? I tell Daddy: It might be a good idea to ask your son to put the books away?

In the following dialogue about Alexandre's bedtime routine, neither of the parents is really listening to the other.

LAZNIK: At the moment it's just a struggle between the two of you and that does not help Alexandre. His bedtime is caught up in the fight between Mummy and Daddy.

MOTHER: Yes, it's a struggle, that's for sure.

I suggest to the mother that she lets the father put his son to bed by himself, while she does something she enjoys – read, watch a film – and trust the father to do his job.

LAZNIK: It would be a pity if we managed to save these wonderful children [from the risk of autism] and then at school they had problems with their behaviour – which has nothing to do with autism! – and try to defy their authority figures, because at home it's Mummy who makes the law.

LAZNIK: Do you know what it's called, this game where we let the father win? It's called femininity. It's a game of 'he who loses, wins'. When we let them win, as fathers, they are all the more loving and attentive towards us.

MOTHER: I understand that, but it's very difficult.

LAZNIK: If you permit me, I will use a few psychoanalytic terms, I don't use to say a lot. [The mother nods.] The mother who 'knows it all' is called the 'phallic' mother. Not only is she the mother – she has given birth to and nursed the baby – but also – she knows! We mothers can feel, we know, and therefore everyone must submit to our knowledge. And first of all, the father, of course, because he does not know. It's very trivial, we're all like that. Then, it's up to us to try and do things differently. But when we are phallic like that, we lose our femininity.

MOTHER: I lay down my arms. I say – ok, that's the intelligent thing to do.

LAZNIK: But in this game of 'he who loses, wins', we are the winners! We win our femininity and their love.

I speak with them about the danger for little boys whose mothers embody the law and who, when they start school, try to defy all kinds of other authorities – teachers, principals ... When the mother can give the father his rightful place, biting her tongues if need be, it seems to work almost like magic. In the days that follow, the problems at school disappear.

FATHER TO THE MOTHER: I'm soaking up Mrs Laznik's words. *The mother laughs.*

I repeat what I had told Patrick's father, some years previously: 'On a boat, there is only one captain and his deputy; this way, the little ones can grow up as little ship's boys.'

We carried them in our womb; if we also want to be the law, the situation turns into a duel, because there is no triangulation, I tell the mother.

MOTHER: Ok, so I bake the cakes, change the nappies and wait for the father's authority?

LAZNIK: You can also make yourself pretty, as you know how to do.

MOTHER: And if I have an idea that the child needs a prohibition at a particular moment. Do I need to hand it over to the father?

Laznik says to the mother that this is the way the Queen, Snow White's step-mother, commands her servant to go and kill.

MOTHER: That's not a very rewarding role.

Laznik explains that a child cannot submit to an authority unless he has first seen an adult doing so.

LAZNIK: A mother can say that this is not her opinion, but that we will do what the father has said.

MOTHER: So the mother's role is never to set prohibitions other than those of the father?

LAZNIK: In a lesbian couple, it is the woman who has not carried the child who is in the role of the third.

MOTHER, SPEAKING TO THE FATHER: Do you realise what a responsibility you have?

The mother wonders if this is why her own parents split up, because her mother always knew better than the father what was good for her children and the father had had enough of it. She says that compared to her own father, her husband is rather docile. He lets her do what she wants. Laznik points out that it is difficult for a father to oppose the phallic maternal power of the mother who knows.

FATHER: All the more so, because in our situation my wife's maternal instinct was kind of broken because of our son Alexandre's illness. I'm sure that when my wife says: 'he's docile, he lets me do what I want, etc.' it's also that I try not to hurt her, because she has already been so hurt by our older son's autism.

LAZNIK: That's a very fine observation. Some specialists say that children who overcome the risk of autism become psychotic. That's not at all necessarily the case. It's simply that sometimes the parents are so paralyzed by the pain they have experienced that instead of doing things as they would have done had the baby not been ill, they are afraid of hurting their partner.

BOTH PARENTS ACQUIESCE: That's it.

LAZNIK: It's very interesting what we're talking about together. When we give fathers their rightful place as fathers, they are very happy with us.

At this moment the baby, who has been sleeping during most of the session, decides to wake up. We explain to him, in simple terms, what the parents have been speaking about.

The baby is no longer completely withdrawn, but still shows difficulties in engaging in the playful exchanges with his mother. The mother in fact has a tendency to rush in communicating with this very sensitive baby and the baby cannot tolerate this. This kind of problem only exists among babies who have an innate excess of emotional empathy and thus find themselves at risk of autism (Laznik, 2014).

Ten days later, the mother and baby finally manage to play together, a game that engages the entire oral drive. The baby offers his little finger to the mother, who finds it delicious; the baby is watching her enraptured and again offers her his little finger. This is a turning point. Everyone is very touched, because we know that for precisely those babies who later become autistic, playing this entire game of the drive is impossible (Laznik, 2009).[3] After the session, as I leave to warm up the baby's bottle, the person filming the session asks the mother what may have caused such a tremendous change. It is true that on that day, the mother approaches the baby much more slowly, responding appropriately to the signs he is giving her. The mother thinks for a while.

MOTHER: Even the session of questioning our parental role, the place of the father and the mother, it had something to do with it. What [the analyst] asked me to do with my son[4] is something that I do not do as a woman. It is all connected, from the boo-boo to the sleepless nights, it is all connected.

Two sessions later, the mother begins to cry. I offer her an individual session that same evening. It turns out that on her way to the session the father told she was just a 'façade'. She thinks this is true. The mother's style has always been slightly hypomanic, which also helped her deal with the fact of having one son on the autistic spectrum and another one who was not yet out of the danger zone. In the following weeks, an entire family history emerges, painful and stretching across generations, a history she was carrying unbeknownst to herself. This gives the mother much more confidence in herself, a confidence that will in turn help her make a bit more room for the father.

Shortly after, Ulysse becomes able to sleep in his own bed. The parents attribute this change to the fact of him not being in quite so much pain anymore, thanks to the work with the osteopath. That is no doubt true. However, the 'questioning' session, as the mother calls it, has perhaps also played a role. The father is finally able to let his voice be heard and is grateful to his wife for letting him make decisions. He organises a surprise weekend for both of them in a luxury spa. It is a success.

As the mother says, it is all connected.

Let me repeat that the children's risk of autism had nothing to do with the mother's difficulty in letting the father play his role; however, it would have been a pity if these boys were later to present with antisocial behaviour.

It so happened that this session brought together several distinct threads. The difficulty of making a place for the paternal function is a phenomenon common to both our clinic and to today's society at large. It has nothing to do with autism, but it can lead to disordered behaviour among children, who subsequently tend to defy social norms. The transgenerational work which the mother was able to carry out in her own sessions, after the father's remark, only made her stronger and gave her a clearer sense of her own history. The same kind of work is also undertaken by all those who, like ourselves, wish to work as psychotherapists. It is rare for a mother to decide to do so, but in this case she did and was the better for it. She will only be a better co-therapist to her baby, considered at a high risk because of his autistic older brother.

What this dialogue between baby Ulysse's parents teaches us is that the difficulty that many fathers in our society have in assuming the paternal function has its roots in the earliest months of the baby's life. Its symptoms can be seen more quickly in boys, because a number of them have problems accepting the social order as soon as they start maternity school.

However, if this difficulty for fathers to carry out their function for their young children is a more general one, what happens to those children who do not present any such symptoms at school? Some Lacanian authors have tried to ask this question in societal terms. Charles Melman (2005) has argued that the 'decline of the *nom du père*' is responsible for the rise in a certain kind of nationalism, leading to a xenophobia against those who are not part of the same nation. A form of 'fatherland' would thus be compensating for the shortcomings of the paternal function. After all, 'fatherland' has to do with the father. A sad solution indeed.

Notes

1 This text has been translated from French, in which the word égalité, here rendered as 'equality', can be interpreted as both parity ('gender equality') and sameness (i.e., a lack of differentiation between the two parental functions). The author's remark warns against this potential confusion.
2 These specialists carry out André Bullinger's sensory-motor assessments, which are essential for the work of a psychoanalyst trying to resuscitate a baby at risk of autism.
3 This hypothesis has been studied on more than 4000 babies. The PREAUT grid has been published in *PLOS ONE* in December 2017. See Olliac et al. (2017).
4 I would often ask her to be more attuned to the signs of this very fragile baby.

Chapter 12

Freud on fathers

Who cares?

Björn Salomonsson

The father according to Freud

Apropos Kai von Klitzing

This chapter contains my points of view – subsumed under five themes – on the various chapters of the book. The first theme summarises the views on fatherhood of 'the Father' himself, that is, Sigmund Freud. I will argue that such an outline, beyond being of historical interest, can illustrate the complex answers to the question, 'What is a father?' Kai von Klitzing (Chapter 2) divides his thoughts on this question into three areas; the father *qua* real father, *qua* part of the parent-child triad, and *qua* internal object. He repeats, as do other authors (Diamond, 2017; Freeman, 2008) and in this volume, for example, Yael Segal, the critique against early psychoanalytic theory; it attributed a restricted role to the father and saw him mainly as a figure that threatens the child's libidinal/dyadic wish to come close to mother. According to Eizirik (2015, p. 343), Freud wrote mainly about the 'the historical oedipal father, the object of desire, or a figure arousing destructive rivalry'. To exemplify, the main character in *Totem and Taboo* (Freud, 1913) is the dead/absent father, far from the man of today accompanying his partner to the antenatal clinic.

Now, is this a fair and complete picture of Freud's view of fatherhood? If not, who cares, a century later? In my view, and here my emphasis differs slightly from Kai's, Freud also recognised another function of the father. True, he thought of it as containing the mother's anxieties and thus helping her respond to the infant's needs, as Kai states in agreement with Britton (1989). But, Freud also suggested that the father *helps the child directly with containment*. I believe that once we recognise this other function, we get a more complete picture of the father's roles (note the plural) – in Freud's *anno dazumal* views and our own of today. Michael J. Diamond (2017) has brought my attention to a passage, where Freud (1930a) states that he 'cannot think of any need in childhood as strong as the need for a father's protection' (p. 72). What kind of father is he speaking of here, and what is it that he must protect the child from? In an earlier treatise on religion, Freud (1927) had spoken of man's illusion of an omniscient, omnipotent, and punishing figure epitomised in the prayer, *Our father who art in heaven*. But in the later work (1930a), the infant is said to need a father for yet another reason; to be protected from the threat against its 'oceanic feeling'. Freud defines this as a 'sensation of "eternity", a feeling as of something limitless, unbounded' (p. 64). The father's task, in the child's mind, is thus to restore 'limitless narcissism' (p. 72). What is at stake here is 'the feeling of infantile helplessness' (p. 72) and thence the child's need for father's protection. This kind of father is very remote from the forbidding and punishing Oedipal father.

Freud, the religious sceptic, did not recognise any oceanic feeling in himself. But he did acknowledge that a 'primary ego-feeling' (Freud, 1930a, p. 68) resides in every human being. It corresponds to a 'more intimate bond between the ego and the world about it' and is thus the affective counterpart to his concept of primary narcissism (Freud, 1914c). Where does it stem from? Clearly, from the infantile period during which Freud indeed gives the father a prominent function of a guardian: The 'terrifying impression of helplessness in childhood aroused the need for protection ... through *love*, which was provided by the father' (Freud, 1927, p. 30, italics added). This helplessness is not only related to the Oedipus complex but begins even earlier with the perceived threat to the primary ego-feeling or narcissism. In *Totem and taboo* (Freud, 1921) Freud adds that the father must have 'equal love' towards every member of the 'primal horde'. If not, 'the family as a natural group formation' will fail to demonstrate its 'indestructible strength' (p. 125). This shows the father's important role in the family's cohesion, not only through his prohibitions but also through his *love*.

Why has Freud's view of the father as patron – a word stemming from *father* – against helplessness been overshadowed by the other perception, that of the father who penalises incest? One answer is that the latter conception receives much greater attention in Freud's writings on the Oedipus complex. Second, the protective father emerges most often in writings that do not focus on development but on religion and anthropology – areas where Freud must remain more speculative and without providing clinical examples. Third, his conception of the infant's helplessness, though hinted at many times from 1895 (Freud, 1950 [1895]) and onwards (Salomonsson, 2018b), was elaborated more clearly rather late (Freud, 1925–6). Fourth, maybe all of us in this profession with 'two rather frightened people: the patient and the psycho-analyst' (Bion, 1990, p. 5) look for a kind of father figure who admonishes us what to do and not to do. Such a proscribing character certainly exists in Freud's writings. When we get caught up in a transference/countertransference gridlock, we may resort to praying for such a figure – and it certainly is easy to find him in Freud's texts. But it is interesting that Freud's other theme, where he suggested that the infant needs the father to allay his/her primal fears, has been in the background for so long in the literature.

Beneath Freud's maritime metaphor 'oceanic feeling', we discern a fantasy about life in the womb. There, every need was fulfilled and no wishful fantasy was needed or even possible. This illusion was smashed to pieces during delivery when the infant was introduced to the rhythm of need and satisfaction, distress and pleasure. Thus arose his/her helplessness as well as the need of a – yes, what? To use von Klitzing's terms, was it the real father, the member of the parent-child triad, or the internal paternal object? I think Freud would have answered, 'In the beginning, it's a mix of the real object and its unconscious representation'.

Must it then be a real man who takes up the protector's role? I agree with Kai: no, a lesbian partner, a grandfather, even a dead father can function as the 'paternal' protector against infantile helplessness. Such alternatives were not addressed by Freud. If we extend the concept of the unconscious father representation to encompass a father *principle*, we realise that the mother herself could, indeed should, entertain this function. The main thing is that this principle is represented in her mind solidly and with a reasonably worked through ambivalence. This is portrayed by a mother who, gently and firmly, can tell the baby: 'No dear, you had your milk, the diaper's changed, I need some time for myself, it's time to sleep. Goodnight'. True, it may be of enormous relief if a real father or partner can help her set limits and assist the baby in coming to terms with his panic. Another gift from the partner is to remind her about the sensual pleasures of the sexual encounter, intertwined as they are with the joys of procreation. As Kai von Klitzing reminds us, 'the origins of life have something to do with sexuality' – in flesh and in fantasy.

Apropos Marie-Christine Laznik

It will come as no surprise that the sexual theme is taken up by a French analyst, Marie-Christine Laznik (Chapter 11, this volume). I had a good laugh when I read about the boy's father's struggle with his disbelief of the therapist. Marie-Christine suggests that his wish to be nice and friendly with his son in fact lies behind the boy's invention of a much worse imago than his father could imagine; the giant and all-destructive monster. The father associates to the movie '*Airplane'*, one of my favourite comic movies. It is about an airplane where all pilots get food-poisoned and unable to fly. The only possible replacement is a passenger; a phobic, impotent, and self-centred man who once was an air force pilot, but whose guilt feelings have made him unable to fly again. He is thus an apt portrait of Patrick's father; nice, benevolent – but haunted by his ghosts in the nursery and thus with little ability to represent the father principle. As Marie-Christine remarks, such men want to share in the maternal care, but it 'does not make one more of a father. A good dad, yes – but not a father'. Linking to Freud's discussions of the father's roles, this father focuses on preserving the boy's belief in the reality of the oceanic experience – but he forgets to personify the guardian of reality and law. The child is thus swaddled in a cocoon of illusions.

When Marie-Christine utilises military metaphors and reminds the father that he does not need to be a 'screaming sergeant' but a captain on board, he divulges that he experienced his own father precisely in this way. I recognise this pattern in many men whom I meet at the Child Health Centre. Similar wishes, not to be like their own father, were also expressed by fathers of new-born's in a qualitative study (Stavrén-Eriksson, 2016): 'More is expected of a modern dad today, when it comes to involvement in the children's upbringing, housework, in everything like that … I think that the dads born in the 40's have missed out on quite a lot' (p. 4). I guess the load which modern fathers experience does not emanate from their fathers' absence or lack of involvement. I rather think that, for a multitude of reasons, they are bewildered or fearful in defining the paternal role, which they do in a negative way: 'I do *not* want to become a father like my dad was'. Since they experienced him as representing No, whether through his absence or prohibitions, and they say No to this ancient figure, the result is a *No to the No* – which is not identical to a *Yes*. They become hyper-tolerant towards their child's demands, an attitude they idealise with formulations such as, 'I do not want to disturb the development of his attachment' or, 'Our family sleeps in the same bed to promote the children's sense of security'. Needless to say, the result is not a secure attachment or agreeable family life but frustration and quarrels. Also, some of these men do resemble the unwilling replacement pilot in '*Airplane*'. They are fearful and feel they have lost control and direction in that life-long flight called parenthood. Or, to use another metaphor, they fail to realise that it is not enough to help the child preserve his oceanic feeling. They must also help the child build a boat and become the captain of the ship of his/her life.

Fathers and sex

Apropos Abel Fagin

We will now enter a field of three agents: the child, the mother and the father. Its many enigmas can be summarised in the formula: 1 + 1 = 3. The greatest mystery of all is: What makes the merger of one plus one result into someone coming from nowhere to pose the great questions: 'Where do I come from? They did it, but how? Will I do it some day?' We now add another role of the father, beyond safeguarding the child's oceanic feeling and forbidding incest; the sexual agent. Male sexuality is also reflected, from a more personal angle, by Abel Fagin (Chapter 8, this volume). He investigates what it means to be a male therapist in a profession dominated by women, and where the parent(s) who seek help expect(s) to see a female therapist. I smile in recognition of my own professional situation … I think many male colleagues would be excellent parent-infant therapists, but they hesitate due to embarrassment, unfamiliarity, and perhaps a fear of being overwhelmed by the sensuous impact in the parent-infant psychotherapy (PIP) session. This brings us to a topic that Abel acknowledges, in junction with Tessa Baradon's chapter; the unspoken sexuality in the room. He notes that it may emerge in the varying transferential ways that mothers, fathers, and babies may experience him. Further, he lists the many countertransference issues that can pop up; sexual attraction, shame, and imprisonment in roles imposed on him by the parent(s).

The contrast between reading the honest and incisive list of the perils and possibilities of being a male therapist, and my waiting for clinical examples, make me wonder: Could it be that although we psychodynamic therapists are trained to acknowledge sexuality as an ever-present part of psychic life, yet have difficulties in doing it fully and without embarrassment? A second question: Are such challenges confined to constellations with a male therapist? Regarding the first question, I bring in Sophie, a one-and-a half-year-old girl who flirts with Abel and finally kisses him while rejecting mother's invitations. Personally, I am less prone to enter into a relationship that is 'child-led and facilitating for the infant [and where] the therapist may initiate and receive appropriate touch, exploration and closeness to take place'. Neither am I certain that this was an 'intimate moment' between the mother, the girl, and Abel. I would rather emphasise another alternative in Fagin's text; by kissing him, the girl avoids intimacy with mother and/or sets up an oedipal rivalry situation. I speculate; what would have happened if Abel had uttered a friendly and unequivocal 'No thank you' to Sophie's kiss? He submits many plausible interpretations of how mother and daughter might experience the kiss and the girl's refusal to kiss Mum. Yet, the main point in exercising the paternal function is to set up boundaries – and to contain the helplessness that is bound to follow. This is why I, when engaging in PIP, generally refrain from touching the infant.

As for the concept of infantile sexuality, recent years have seen its revival (Laplanche, 2002; Widlöcher, 2002), and the recognition of its impact from infancy to adulthood (Salomonsson, 2012; Stein, 1998; Zamanian, 2011; Zeuthen & Gammelgaard, 2010). These investigations have redefined it, from an abstruse force leaning onto (Freud, 1905) the instinct of survival to a steady and ever-present current in every human interaction. If we place a therapist or parent of any gender in this constellation, we grasp the impact s/he may have on the relationship between mother and baby. This is where Fagin, and Baradon, focus their investigations. Whatever the gender of the therapist, it yields different experiences for the mother and the father in treatment. Various emotions may surge; hetero-/homo-erotic attraction, shame, jealousy, dyadic bliss, triangular exclusion, anger, contempt ... Fagin's and Baradon's point is that this hot spot should be investigated in every PIP therapy.

To briefly answer my second question, if these issues revolve only around male therapists, I would say no. The gender homogeneity among pre- and post-natal health care nurses and PIP therapists can lure us into thinking that it is a no-sex area. Though this is true in a manifest sense, on a latent level it is not. This was Freud's point when he argued that

> no one who has seen a baby sinking back satiated from the breast and falling asleep with flushed cheeks and a blissful smile can escape the reflection that this picture persists as a prototype of the expression of sexual satisfaction in later life.
>
> (Freud, 1905, p. 182)

Infantile sexuality is 'everywhere' in the sense that we think and experience our world, not only with our thinking head but also with our lust-seeking body. This goes for therapists and our patients as well, and the deeper we realise it, the better we can help them.

Apropos Joan Raphael-Leff

My mind veers to another aspect on fatherhood and sexuality apropos Joan Raphael-Leff (Chapter 6, this volume). She quotes Freud (1939) as he discusses the societal shift from emphasising the mother to the father. This

> points in addition to a *victory of intellectuality over sensuality* – that is, an advance in civilization, since maternity is proved by the evidence of the senses while paternity is a hypothesis, based on an inference and a premiss. Taking sides in this way with a *thought-process* in preference to a sense perception has proved to be a momentous step.
>
> (pp. 113–14, italics added)

This is similar to Lacan's discussion of the adage that Freud (1909c) had referred to earlier: *Pater semper incertus est, mater certissima est.* The father is always uncertain, the mother is very certain. This insecurity has forced humanity to create laws, family bonds, and abstract thinking, as Freud suggests.

To nullify fatherhood is to attack the basic principles of society – and abstract thinking itself. This also helps us understand the worries that many men face when approaching fatherhood; it is such an abstract undertaking! Talking about salaries, cars, ski resorts, even sex is no big deal compared with broaching the mysterious topic of fatherhood: 'What am I to expect, how will I experience it, what kind of father will I become one day?' The woman is helped by her bodily changes to grasp what it may mean to become a parent. In a qualitative study, Genesoni & Tallandini (2009) portray men's dilemmas in their transition to fatherhood. They view themselves as part of a 'labouring couple' and join their partner in midwifery exams, etc. They do want to bond emotionally with the future child but – and this is a problem arising from their 'incertus' position – they also suffer from 'feelings of unreality, arising out of the lack of tangible evidence of the existence of their unborn child' (p. 313). They struggle with being outsiders and also feel they must be strong and supportive of the partner and that their worries are minor compared with hers (Stavrén-Eriksson, 2016).

Joan suggests, and this differs from my position, that 'our parenting responses are not instinctively predetermined by biology or imprinting'. I would emphasise that the responses are not *only* biologically or ecologically predetermined. We can never know to what extent societal roles or gender patterns determine that a father ends up in one of the categories that she has coined, for example, the 'Renouncer' or 'Participator'. But we do know that he cannot run away from the fact that 'anatomy is destiny' (Freud, 1912). I give full credit to the many critics of Freud's lopsided and incomplete theory of the psychological impact of the differences between the sexes. Nevertheless, we should beware of throwing out the baby with the bathwater – not the least when it comes to discussing fatherhood. Our parenting responses are not only instinctively predetermined by biology or imprinting, since they also depend on our capacity to 'question psycho-historical meanings'. And, we can and should 'attempt to improve on them', as Joan suggests. But these efforts will also meet with an absolute limit; it takes two gametes to make a child; one must come from a man and one from a woman, and only the latter's body will carry the child – while the man remains an outsider. For example, when newly pregnant women declared in an interview study (Bergbom, Modh, Lundgren, & Lindwall, 2016) that 'their body had longed to become pregnant and have children and now they felt a sense of bodily fulfilment' (p. 582), it would be absurd if such a statement were expressed by their male partner. What I am defending here is the impact of biological limitations, from which both sexes suffer. But, if the protagonists handle these facts humbly and with fascination, they can also thrive on these differences.

Apropos Yael Segal

Yael Segal is also into sexuality, focusing on what may happen between a female therapist and a male patient/father (Chapter 9, this volume). Adult sexuality is expressed more clearly in her second vignette through the father's erotic text messages. Her apprehension of being 'harassed' blinds her and she cannot discern that behind his flirts, a man is hiding who is terrified of taking responsibility of a baby boy whose mother is schizophrenic. Her first case has some similarities in that she meets with a father, whose prominent masculinity evokes memories of her own and often absent father. Here, too, such forces blind her from seeing the help-seeking appeals behind the man's assertive behaviour.

Macho-like behaviour has different repercussions on a female and a male therapist, respectively. A woman may rightly fear harassment, as Yael did initially in her second case. As a male PIP therapist, I have also met many assertive fathers. This often reflects various defences; the man may feel dragged by his wife to me to be rectified for his sloppy behaviour qua father. He may thus feel backstabbed even before our first encounter. In addition, he may experience me via a father-like transference position and fear that I will belittle him. If the wife then casts an appreciative glance at me, the scene is set for a jealousy drama.

Segal's two cases show how infantile and adult sexuality blend imperceptibly in therapeutic encounters. She fears the text-message-sending man's advances – and she also interprets them along the tracks of her unconscious sexuality; men are big, enticing, and dangerous. This is portrayed in an even more moving way when she relates, in the first case, that the father 'brought into the room a wave of strong manhood, with the unmistakable smell of military laundry'. When we hear, later, about her own father, an army officer, we understand the lifelong impact of these smells in her mind. We also see the beauty of therapeutic work when a therapist, via the insight about such unconscious forces, manages to liberate herself and becomes freer to navigate and help the father.

Still, there is one point of disagreement between Segal and me. She criticises the tendency among therapists and their theories 'to prioritise the exclusive mother-infant relationship [which has] has deep roots in our culture' (Chapter 9, this volume). I would add that this relationship is also rooted in our *bodies*. The formula 1 + 1 = 3 does not merely imply, as Kai von Klitzing suggests, that 'the origins of life have something to do with sexuality'. It also tells us that the origins of the infant's *mind* have something to do with sexuality; it is born inside, and then outside, the mother. The concept of a 'fatherhood constellation', which Segal speaks of, has the same amount of validity as does 'the motherhood constellation'. But in the beginning, the former constellation has a more abstract and less corporal anchorage than that of the motherhood constellation. I agree with Yael that 'the birth of a baby can undermine the father's male identity'. In my experience, one way of helping such men is to point out that female and male constellations are different. 'Now it's mother's time, and soon it'll be yours', as I sometimes tell a bewildered and unassuming father. This can give rise to envy, mourning, jealousy, impatience – but also to love, relief, and a stronger sense of masculinity.

Fathers and the triad

Apropos Tessa Baradon

After having discussed Fagin's and Segal's cases, we realise the complexity and the challenges implied in PIP. When someone decides to start therapy training, s/he may choose between becoming a couple/child/adult/individual or group therapist. But, in the domain of *parent-infant* therapy the therapist needs to be specialized in all these areas. Not only are all these foci involved in such work but there is also a constant switch between them. Switches may occur from one session to another; a mother may come alone for the first session to complain at length about her depression. One word about the baby's distress may alert the therapist, who then suggests her to bring the child to the next session. Individual work thus has become dyadic. She may then voice bitterness towards her spouse, and he gets invited for the third session. Now, they're into 'working with the triad', which is Tessa Baradon's focus in Chapter 7 of this volume.

Already her quotation by Stern shows Tessa's intention to look at every participant in her consulting room from a systems theory perspective (Emde, 1988; Sander, 2002; von Bertalanffy, 1968). This implies to understand that each participant in a session takes on a role according to which place(s) s/he occupies – for the moment – in that grand system called 'the family'. For example, a man turned father may suddenly experience shifts in his identity, position, responsibilities, and emotions vis-à-vis himself, his partner, parents, siblings, workmates, and the baby. The woman, until now his girlfriend, is now his companion parent. His father, previously a distant figure, has now become a colleague in parenthood. Thus, no man can be studied without taking into account the networks he is involved in and the roles he is assuming. This makes working with the triad utterly complicated, especially since Tessa also studies each member from, if I may, a 'non-systems theory' perspective. As a child/individual therapist, she never forgets the human being with his/her past history and present fantasy world.

Baradon's point is to constantly monitor the therapeutic process in PIP with a binocular focus; she seeks out what happens in the individual subject, be it the baby, mother or father: 'How is mother today? How did the baby react when mother started crying or when father made an ironic comment?' Tessa's other focus implies to scan what goes on within the group qua system: 'Why does this family, who went through such ghastly things recently, seem so well-ordered?' (The examples are mine). Sometimes, this shift between the two foci gets implemented in a change of setting that Tessa calls 'irregular arrangements'. I would add that such shifts often occur on a minute-to-minute basis in the session. The case of Lila and her family is a case to the point. In addition to addressing little Lila's crankiness, Tessa obviously wants to engage her father, a despondent and passive immigrant, in being a parent. He responds to her invitation and picks up a toy train to draw Lila's attention. This is a moment of father-daughter therapy. Some minutes later, Tessa picks up his choice of the train to indicate his solitude and helplessness as a 'passenger' into the UK. Now, we are into his individual therapy. But, since he is also told that the train indicates his wish to protect Lila, the intervention also focuses on the father-daughter relationship. Finally, when mother listens to this interchange with compassion, yet another focus is included; the triad. From this vertex, she becomes a partner who gets to understand his plight better.

Taken together, the many components of Tessa's 'train' intervention illustrate that her term 'working with the triad' can be compared to reading a musical partition; if we read it cross-sectionally, we can focus on one part at a time; which tone is played right now by the clarinet, the strings, and the brass? Or, we can imagine how all these notes might sound together. If read longitudinally, we can see the development over time; how does the first theme die out to be replaced by the second? The PIP therapist thus works like a conductor who overhears and maintains contact with each musician. Tessa, an experienced *chef d'orchestre*, summarises that she supported 'father's and baby's agency in reaching out to each other' and helped them 'join up'. Her bridging these two parts/voices presupposed that she listened to a third part as well: She also tuned in to the muted cry of father's solitude, which she overheard and brought out by suggesting what the train might symbolise to *him* personally. He thus got in contact with his pain, which helped him console his daughter. Beautiful polyphonic music!

Baradon then moves on to addressing the therapist's 'paternal function', 'a reflective mind that enables simultaneous containment of the mother-infant dyad and their separateness'. I think (Salomonsson, 1998), like others do (Maiello, 2007; Quinodoz, 1992; see also Chapter 11, this volume), that we can differentiate between two grand worldviews and modes of relating; the maternal and the paternal. This is pure Lacan (1998b). A father who, like in the trainee's report, exclaims when seeing his baby fondling mother's breasts, 'Hey, those breasts are mine', is executing the paternal function. To get back to Freud and fathers, this father appears as the guardian against incest. He introduces the law and the word, and thus draws a line between infantile and adult sexuality, or between boundless pleasure and lust combined with responsibility. In contrast, I am not so sure that 'containment of the mother-infant dyad' represents that same paternal function. If a father listens to and empathises with his partner's woes and their baby's crying, I claim that he is executing, paradoxical as it may sound, a maternal containment; he identifies with and attends specifically to her motherly worries.

Should we then skip the sexual epithets of the two kinds of containment we are discussing? Should we regard such labels as outdated prejudices that merely reflect our projections about the two genders? Yet, as I already argued, and as Tessa reminds us now, there is a sexual presence in every family with a baby. Or, to quote Kai von Klitzing again, 'the origins of life have something to do with sexuality'. Tessa she reminds us that we tend to repress the sexuality inherent in PIP work, simply because it is so brazen. As she puts it, when the therapist meets with 'the fluids, odours, excretions, mess, appetite and emotional vehemence – [they are] all evocative of (the recent) intercourse'. Such connections are rarely addressed by the parents, or the therapist presenting a case, for that matter. Whether they will be addressed by the therapist in the session depends on his/her perception of the present moment, attitudes to sexuality, personal experiences, etc. But, if s/he remains deaf to these signals, many parts of the musical score will remain muted, and the treatment will remain an unfinished symphony. I think such deafness can negatively affect the therapeutic outcome.

Apropos Louise Emanuel

How does the child experience all this 'sex stuff'? To answer, we can turn to Louise Emanuel (Chapter 10, this volume), which is necessarily brief due to her sad and untimely demise. It demonstrates how she, a post-Kleinian therapist, assumed that unconscious fantasies exist in a young child. Her examples also demonstrate that the interpretations of such fantasy content were founded on detailed observations of the child's behaviour in the therapy room. Maria, two-and-a-half years old, draws circles and hands them to the adults in a 'teacher-like' manner. Whereas the mother attributes this to Maria's preschool teachings, Emanuel thinks she shows her need to be in the centre rather than being marginalised in the corner of an Oedipal triangle. It is as if she were signalling: 'OK, you claim the origins of life have something to do with sexuality. If so, I wanna be part of that secret confederacy!' Louise bases her interpretation on the assumption that a circle symbolises eternal dyadic bliss while an edgy triangle corresponds to exclusion. Such thinking follows the Kleinian agenda of attributing to children, even younger ones than Maria, capacities of symbolising their struggles with internal and external objects. Though many analysts have been critical towards Klein's conclusions, Emanuel has one trump card to support her thesis. The fact that Maria steadily avoids looking at *her* she interprets, correctly as I see it, to indicate that the girl is suspicious of Louise's intentions of destabilising the family structure. Indeed, that is Louise's aim.

What has this got to do with fathers and the paternal function? Emanuel, as do some other authors in this volume, uses the terms paternal and maternal functions as a matter of course. The paternal function implies a benign but firm boundary and limit setting, a capacity for 'penetrative' insight, and the courage to come up with new ideas and initiatives. (But, let us not forget Freud's complementary view of the father who helps the child cope with the threats against the oceanic feeling). The maternal implies to tenderly receive a child's communications of pleasure and distress. Emanuel emphasises that the two do not indicate specific qualities in men and women, respectively, a point I raised briefly earlier. Instead, they need to coexist in *both* parents to establish a well-functioning couple. In Maria's family, however, the paternal function seems compromised in both parents: in the father, by his readiness to get out of bed and spend hours with the sleepless daughter in her room; in the mother, by replacing her wedding ring with Maria's plastic ring. This paves the way for confusion and omnipotence in the girl, who ascends from princess to pseudo-queen.

When Maria avoids looking at Emanuel, I think it is mostly the paternal aspect of containment that she fears. I see this as a negative transference expressed in a fantasy like 'This woman tries to take me away from Mum and Dad, whom I love and control. I demand bribes, I hand out circle drawings, and their bedroom is also *my* property and queendom'. Thus, though this father does not seem to have any vast personal problems, the family certainly has issues with the paternal function. And this is, precisely, what Emanuel tries to help them with, obviously with quite good results.

The breakdown of fatherhood and transgenerational trauma

Apropos Angela Joyce

A father's ability to represent the paternal function obviously depends on his relationships, internal and external, with own his parents – perhaps most conspicuously with his father. Angela Joyce (Chapter 3, this volume) and Amanda Jones (Chapter 5, this volume) bring up fathers for whom such relationships were brittle and agonising, which also darkened their relationships with the baby and the spouse. We are thus into the topic of the *telescoping of transgenerational trauma* (Faimberg, 1988). The basic idea that we are affected by the internal worlds of our forefathers was introduced notably by Ferenczi (1933). The point is that the scars of previous generations remain secret or even taboo and thus, the next generation can neither face it openly nor integrate it (Mészáros, 2010). Faimberg formulates the tricky clinical question thus: How can the therapist and the patient talk about something, which the patient does not think concerns him and the analyst is ignorant of?

In PIP, it may take much meandering before such a previous and buried trauma is revealed. The point of departure in Angela Joyce's case is a mother who has suffered a traumatic delivery and whose son is agitated and screaming. The father is described as merely fulfilling the clichés of an unhelpful husband. In PIP work, such complaints sometimes cover up a severe marital conflict, the mother's struggle with guilt feelings and a faltering self-esteem, etc. But here, as Joyce discovers, the father really *is* weighed down by problems. They stem from events way back in life, and they affect not only his capacities as a husband but also as a father. Memories of having lost his parents in childhood are knocking on the door when he himself becomes a father. Just about when he has become a colleague with his parents he discerns, vaguely and against heavy resistance, that he cannot tell them about this momentous event simply, but not merely, because they are deceased. This awakens pain in him; both present and ancient. It is perhaps to overstretch the concept of transgenerational transmission in father Andrew's case, since he knew about the deaths of his parents. But, he did not link his vague paternal role with the losses he had failed to mourn and come to terms with. Therefore, had this theme not been approached in therapy, he might have created a transgenerational trauma for his son Tommy – for example, by not recognising his importance for the boy and by 'pushing him to keep achieving, driving forward, not relaxing'.

A technical issue emerges in Angela's chapter: Who is the patient; mother a/o baby a/o father (Baradon, Salomonsson, & von Klitzing, 2014)? In her presentation, we discover that this cannot be answered once and for all. Rather, she needs to focus, from session to session, on which participant(s) has (have) the sorest spot. This challenges her countertransference; as soon as she decided to focus on the father's repressed memories and pain, she felt she was leaving behind the depressed mother Rosie and little Tommy. Joyce argues that her reaction reflected 'the defensive wall that Andrew had created around his childhood losses'. I would add that she was *bound* to feel she abandoned them when turning to Andrew's pain and his shoving it 'through the door in the back of his head'. Yet, Rosie did not only feel forsaken by this focus but also felt confirmed in her intuitions that something was the matter with her partner. Her wish to get to know him better was pivotal and gave the therapist leeway to pursue her attention on Andrew. Again, this shows the advantage of, at least at one point or another, having both parents participating in PIP work.

Then comes the finale; a summer break and – as Angela sees it – an interrupted treatment. After having experienced quite a few such 'interruptions' at the Child Health Centre, I have come to reconsider how to interpret them, specifically, by comparing the results with the patients' expectations. We must ask; what were the reasons for this couple to seek therapy? Indeed, it was *not* the father's wish to come to grips with his childhood history but the mother's sadness and the boy's screaming. In this, they got substantial help. Thus, if we place the bar at a level that corresponds to the parents' expectations, they got what they asked for. Were we instead eager to focus on the deaths of his parents, how he defended against the ensuing pain, and how this made him a 'frozen' father, we would have to acknowledge that some thawing did occur in therapy – but not enough. I empathise with, and recognise, Angela's disappointment in the countertransference, but I think this is part and parcel of every PIP therapist's work. Stern (1995) observed that parents with baby worries seldom regard themselves as mentally ill but as being in a crisis or a state of chock. True, the ground may have been brittle due to earlier character problems, neurotic symptoms, and relational frailties. But their defences have functioned reasonably well until now – as in Andrew's case. I think he received as much thawing as he wanted or could manage. One day he may, or may not, opt for more warming up of his emotions and defences. But for now he, and we, have every reason to feel this therapy helped him become a warmer and more accessible father.

Apropos Amanda Jones

The transgenerational theme is addressed explicitly by Amanda Jones (Chapter 5, this volume), which brings out the brutal realities in some families with small children. She speaks of fathers who have little of so many assets; an understanding of their and others' feelings, a wish to learn more about them, and an insight that their own emotional state will affect the mother's well-being and the baby's social and emotional development. Her chapter is thus a healthy reminder that today's proponents of fathers' rights and roles should beware of being naïve. Many modern men declare that they are committed to co-operating with their spouse in creating a healthy and loving environment for the baby. But, as Amanda reminds us, not all of them are willing to submit themselves to the emotional, mutual and hard work that parenthood demands.

Why do some men develop in this direction, and why do some women choose to live with them and have children? In her theorising, Amanda focuses on the second question, I think in a very respectable mission of being the spokeswoman and guardian of mother and baby when a father is a self-centred psychopath. Jones understands 'the magnetic attraction' that some women feel for these men as reflecting an 'illness of transgenerational relational origin'. Indeed, 'it takes many more than two people to make a baby: a group of ghosts may come to the fore'. One such revenant, hiding behind the brutal man, can be the woman's strong and deeply ambivalent relationship with her internal mother imago. Hendrika Freud (2011) has compared this relationship to that of the ancient tragic heroines Electra and her mother Clytemnestra whom she hates – and yearns for. Some women seek, via a destructive relationship with her male sexual partner, to avoid being clutched in the grips of a monstrous version of her mother – only to discover that she is trapped in a second edition of hostile abandonment and, sometimes also, ruthless violence.

To uncover such forces causes suffering for the woman and thence, she may be aversive towards treatment for herself and the baby. Via video recordings and a technique of speaking with the baby's voice, Jones helps mother see these patterns. Her theoretical model focuses, mainly but not merely, on the mother's and, more speculatively, the father's defensive activities. This is 'relational ego psychology' in the post-Anna Freud tradition at its best; intellectually clear and emotionally incisive. Jones gives a credible model of transgenerational influence, which threatens to also hit baby Ben. The mother feels enslaved by her partner, who stands in for her internal parents. This chain is on its way to extend into her relationship with the baby boy. This can be seen when the boy, after the mother's repeated rejections, begins to have a tense face like his mother. One question, impossible to answer for the moment, remains: Is Ben already sliding into the grips of transgenerational affliction – or was this forestalled in therapy? On the positive side, Amanda mentions Ben's resilience, which she attributes to his mother's attention to his physical needs and his siblings' support. True, the prefix 'transgenerational' should thus not mislead us into thinking that influences run along a straight line. We are reminded that many factors can fill in the 'transmission gap' (Fonagy & Target, 2005; van IJzendoorn, 1995).

Fathers and psychotherapeutic technique

Apropos Alejandra Perez

I have already addressed various technical aspects in PIP; the 'irregular arrangements' of changing between dyadic and triadic work, the sexuality in the parents' and the therapist's minds, switching between the parent's present ailment and past haunting history, etc. Alejandra Perez brings in (Chapter 4, this volume), a bit more consistently than the other authors, the baby. True, it is plain to see her sensitivity in capturing and addressing the emotional pain that the two *parents* are struggling with. But beyond that, she focuses on the *baby's* role as catalyst (Fraiberg, 1987) and dialogue partner. I refer to the section 'Waking Daddy up ...', when Oliver is beginning to show an autistic-like state. Despite the therapist's and the parents' efforts at moving on from talking about their unhappy childhood experiences and developing in their parental functions, something is still missing, and this is what Oliver signals; he is unhappy and is distancing himself from the ongoing tension and skirmish.

Such moments when an infant shows distress are of course alarming but also, if handled sensitively on the spot, of enormous value. Perez demonstrates this beautifully when addressing the boy. She asks him if he is looking out of the window because he finds it difficult to hear mummy being upset, and if he feels it is all too much and tries to escape. Alan, the father, reacts promptly by reflecting on similar situations at home, and by asking if the therapist thinks baby Oliver can understand such things. Perez describes this as the father's 'waking up'. One could, with equal justification, claim that *so did Oliver and his mother Celia as well*. When the therapist placed Oliver in the limelight, his distress obviously diminished. This illustrates the point of inviting the baby to sessions. Firstly, because Oliver showed that the parents' strained relationship was not only their business but his as well. Second, when parents perceive their child's 'radar function' of picking up their emotional communication, their concern for the child helps them step out of their regressed state and become aware of his needs and separate existence (cf. when Celia thoughtfully remarks that she has noticed Oliver's staring away at home); this paves the way for a more affectionate behaviour towards him.

One final point: perinatal psychiatric care is sometimes organised in ways that might send signals that 'quick fixes' are possible. I have argued that sometimes, such brief consultations may indeed be of great value (Salomonsson, 2018a). But, we should not fool ourselves into thinking that this is the general rule. The family presented by Perez could not have made any substantial progress without her committed and skilful *long-term* psychotherapeutic work. This also applies to most cases in this volume. In an era saluting rapid but shallow progress, not the least in psychiatry, this needs to be pointed out to politicians and patients. We should be quick in instituting parent-infant therapy, but think twice before terminating it.

Chapter 13

Three themes about fathers in parent-infant psychotherapy

Björn Salomonsson, Tessa Baradon and Kai von Klitzing

This final discussion chapter emerged from the three-way conversations we had as the chapters came in and the book progressed. We realised that particular themes were recurring and 'grabbing our interest'. Transference-countertransference dynamics are commented on by all the contributors – as would be expected in a psychoanalytic book. However, different positions are taken with regards to whether there is a specific form and expression of 'fathers' transference'? This theme is taken up by Björn Salomonsson.

In the clinical chapters various intervention approaches are described. To an extent, each is a co-construction unique to the particular family and therapist, but in some measure, different interventions bear the stamp of the theoretical framework and personal style of each therapist. Tessa Baradon attempts to create schema from the exquisitely personal ways of being and of intervening that the therapists describe in their work with their patients.

We also discussed questions pertaining to triangulation, noting the challenges fathers and mothers face in becoming a triad, and may pass on to their baby. However, what about the therapist's capacities for triadifiction? This topic is discussed by Kai von Klitzing.

ON TRANSFERENCE AND COUNTERTRANSFERENCE *BJÖRN SALOMONSSON*

This section summarises my thoughts on transference and countertransference when working with fathers in parent-infant psychotherapy (PIP). First of all, do such specific phenomena exist at all? If so, what might be their various manifestations and how should we handle them? I will begin by briefly defining the transference concept and proceed to discussing these questions. Some examples will be drawn from the book's clinical cases, and one from my own PIP experiences.

Transference: a working definition

Let us imagine two people talking about the same person, for example, their boss. One says: 'He's wonderful, supportive, warm, and encouraging. He brings out the best in me!' The other: 'He's unpleasant. I never know what he wants from me. Always that frown on his face. I feel belittled by him, always scared I've made a mistake.' True, their boss can act differentially towards them, and they may also have different work tasks and positions in the company, but a psychoanalytic investigation might add that their *transference-like reactions* to the boss are at odds. Some father-like attributes occur in both, the first has a benevolent characteristic, while the other one veers towards a stern and castrating figure.

To explain the term transference, we must first note its various usages among Kleinian and Freudian analysts. They all refer to situations in which unconscious wishes constituted of 'infantile prototypes' (Laplanche & Pontalis, 1973, p. 455) are actualised in the analyst-analysand relationship. This colours the patient's views of the therapist in various unrealistic directions; s/he is idealised, scorned, hated, yearned for, etc. Also, such feelings and attitudes oscillate and change as treatment proceeds. Freud (1912) claimed that we must understand the dynamics of transference, because on this field 'the victory must be won – the victory whose expression is the permanent cure of the neurosis' (p. 108). Today's therapists are less naive in hoping for a 'permanent cure' and know that they must take into account their countertransference as well, that is, the contributions emanating from *their* unconscious. Still, what defines psychodynamic psychotherapies, in whatever settings, and provides the template for their capacity to help the patient, is our understanding of how transferences appear and are to be handled.

Before we focus on fathers' transferences, we need to summarise how Kleinians and Freudians conceive of transference *in general*. Freudians use it in the sense of a *sustained* colouring of an object relation rather than a temporary affect. In contrast, Melanie Klein preferred the broader term 'transference situation' (Petot, 1990, p. 139) referring to all unconscious fantasies 'rooted in the earliest stages of development and in the deep layers of the unconscious' (Klein, 1952, p. 55). Today's contemporary Freudian and Kleinian views have come closer, and both speak of the possibility of transference emerging already in childhood and, also, 'from the outset of the analysis' (Sandler & Sandler, 1994, p. 387). Today's Kleinians (Spillius, 1983) tend to postpone giving transference interpretations until they have performed a detailed analysis of the patient-analyst interaction, including the countertransference perspective. This double focus is implied by the term 'transference as the total situation' (Joseph, 1985).

If we briefly return to the two work-mates' discussion about their boss, we recognise that *transference-like* phenomena operate throughout life and influence all human relations (Klein, 1928, p. 48). The idea of transference is thus an extension of a trivial fact; we can never know our fellow human being 'as he really is', because our perceptions always proceed from our subjectivity. What psychoanalysis has added is that such subjectivity is multi-layered and varies according to the circumstances and periods of life that we and the study object are in for the moment. I have therefore suggested that we 'speak of *transference* only when we can investigate it accurately, that is, in the analytic situation' (Salomonsson, 2013, p. 775).

Transference, countertransference and affects

The section above might be perceived as lopsided were it to define transference as the patient's 'faulty perception' of the therapist. Although this can be true, the therapist must of course scrutinise how s/he may contribute as to how the patient perceives him/her. In other words, s/he must strive to be aware of the interplay between transference and countertransference. Another important factor is to acknowledge the current affects in this interplay. Let us turn to Yael Segal's second case of little Eli and his father (Chapter 9, this volume). He feels reproached by the therapist's judgment and criticism. She does not recognise his need for support because he disguises it behind an erotic parade. She gets angry and aversive, while he becomes anxious and dumbfounded.

With the help of a supervisor she realises that, viewed from the *transference* vantage point, the father sexualises his 'non-sexual' need of her to calm his anxiety. This insight is only possible once the therapist is ready to look at her own aversion towards him. I get the impression that up to this point, her interpretations of the father's behaviour have become stuck; she speaks of his 'infatuation for her', loaded with 'erotic allusions' and of his 'expensive Parker pen' gift being 'a barely disguised phallic symbol'. Viewed from the countertransference vantage point, this creates a stalemate in her functioning. Not until she perceives the depth and extent of the countertransference impact can she become more relaxed towards what she labels his 'urgent erotic need' for her. True, he may display a 'transformed defensive expression of his fear of raising his son alone, without a maternal figure'. But, it can also reflect the father's *maternal* transference, in which he sees the therapist as a good, omnipotent mother who can fix everything and spirit away his sick wife, without his feeling guilty – and perhaps even without having an adult, sexual desire of her.

I brought in the case of Eli's father and the therapist to show that whenever we describe how a patient experiences the therapist, it must remain a sketchy label. There is no such thing as a pure *father* transference, an absolute *negative* transference, etc. The most important lesson from the therapist's supervision in Segal's case is that it increased her 'ability to "read the signs" and understand the dynamics unfolding in the room as well as in her mind'. Thus, when we speak of a father's transference in PIP treatment, we should ask: 'OK, now I discovered this phenomenon, and what may be hiding underneath?' To exemplify this multi-layered system, I will bring in Tessa Baradon, with the immigrant father playing with a train with his eight-month-old daughter Lila (Chapter 7, this volume). Here is a destitute, illegal immigrant who strikes the therapist as 'extremely passive in his parenting endeavour'. It is not difficult to imagine that this man is highly suspicious of Tessa, perhaps experiencing her as a societal controller, as a know-it-all about parenthood, and as a member of that sex who knows best how to take care of children.

I am convinced that Tessa has all these possibilities in mind. She might choose between making such an interpretation or doing what she did; she observed the joint father-daughter play and said to the girl: 'Daddy is driving the train, it is coming clo-s-e-r'. If we are right that he harboured a negative transference, it evidently diminished through her intervention and he became a more active father. The next intervention shows her understanding of a deeper lying transference, something like 'this woman has no clue what it feels like to be an outcast and an illegal immigrant'. But, when Tessa addresses the link between the train and immigration, he becomes more emotional. The transference has now switched from feelings of suspicion and exclusion to warmth, mourning, and inclusion. This example also shows that the important thing may not be to *interpret* the transference, but to *acknowledge* it, a topic I will broach in the next section.

There is another take at the concept of 'the father transference', namely, the baby's transference towards the father. I have written about a therapy with a father and his nine-month-old son Vance (Salomonsson, 2013). The father was about to go on paternal leave with the boy. A restless character, he had indeed been a hyperactive child, he feared he would not be able to bond with his son well enough. Against such premonitions, he upheld a cheerful façade during our first session, claiming that no problems remained now. This contrasted with the boy's panic when looking at me. The next session, father was better prepared to acknowledge that he was also scared of seeing me as a know-it-all mind-reader. This enabled him to reach a more genuine contact with the boy, he could comfort him, and Vance calmed down. Father could then speak more truthfully of his childhood sorrows. I concluded that as long as he muted his own anxiety of being with me, he became threatening to the boy who reacted with distress. When father became more permeable to his fears of me, he transformed into a more comprehensible character to the boy, whose negative transference towards Dad, and secondarily also to me, thus decreased visibly.

This case also showed that all is not father transference that looks like it. Later in therapy, the boy suddenly panicked when he was striding proudly across the room, away from father and me. This particular session took place in another office room than he was used to. I thought of the incident as reflecting the boy's acute separation anxiety and brought up with the father something he had mentioned before but which we had never delved into; two months earlier the family visited the mother's family in her native country. She then returned home while the boy remained there with father. When father and son united with mother, Vance was quiet and sad. So was the mother, but nobody dared speaking about it. It seemed that the boy's panic when walking away from father in the session reflected earlier experiences of separation from mother. We may suggest that for the moment, he had a temporary maternal transference – of a deserting and probably depressive mother – towards his father. As we see once again, transference is a multi-layered phenomenon.

Transference: acknowledging and/or interpreting it?

I stated earlier, when discussing the case of Tessa Baradon's immigrant father that acknowledging the present transference is not equal to suggesting that it should always be interpreted. Let us look at Alejandra Perez's case of baby Oliver and his mother Celia, diagnosed with borderline personality disorder, and his father Alan (Chapter 4, this volume). The father is passive, almost drowsy, while mother is nagging at him in despair. Still, there are some sensitive interchanges with father Alan and son. I would guess that in the countertransference, the therapist must have felt impotent and perhaps angry at seeing a man being, and letting himself be, discarded in his paternal competence and affection. It might be tempting to link this with the mother's complaints towards baby and father in an intervention like: 'I wonder how it feels for you, Alan, when Celia criticises you and feels that Oliver prefers your care to hers'. However, this was not what Alejandra did, because she perceived an 'unreflective family fusion'. Such a construction entails that when the therapist shows signs of having a mind of her own, with different thoughts, she is experienced as intrusive. This paves the way for epistemic mistrust or hypervigilance (Allison & Fonagy, 2016), that is, a suspicion that can 'prevent an individual from sufficiently trusting others to learn from them, [which can be] a major barrier to therapeutic change' (p. 277).

Had Alejandra made the interpretation just mentioned, Celia's mistrust might be awakened, as well as Alan's fear of her. Importantly, the therapist also recognised another reason for Celia's fear of such an intervention. To her, the enmeshed relationship in the couple 'had protected her from an unreliable and abusive world'. Any such intervention would thus constitute a serious threat to this construction. Celia's difficulties in being a mother are portrayed in greater detail elsewhere (Perez, 2018). But, was Celia the only problem? Certainly not. Alan was besieged by guilt, self-punishment, and a defensive effacing of troubling emotions. Thence his meek efforts at resisting when Celia was pestering him.

For different yet confluent reasons, both parents contributed to the boy's passivity and seclusion. Now, if the therapist is advised against making the interpretation mentioned earlier, what should she do to 'wake Daddy up'? Perez's solution was to 'explore and work on the particular triangular relationships and dynamics in the family', yet struggle to maintain the brittle therapeutic alliance with each parent. This sounds good enough, but how to do it? As it often happens in PIP work, the baby came up with the answer. With dazed, absent eyes, Oliver looked out of the window as Mum complained about her depression. The therapist now addressed the boy, suggesting it was all too much for him and that he was trying to escape. This awakened father's interest and he voiced similar concerns from home. Oliver became enlivened, and so did Celia's contact with him. Thus, in an indirect way, with no explicit transference interpretation being uttered, this father came to understand that his passivity, guilt, and fear of his wife did have a negative effect on the boy. What I find interesting and admirable is that this technique – being aware of the parents transferences without necessarily voicing them explicitly – lead to changes in both of them: 'Celia allowing [the baby] to separate, and Alan being more present'. Evidently, there was another beneficiary, too: Little Oliver became more enterprising and more in contact with both parents.

Whereas Perez's case shows some reasons why being too explicit too early about the transference can affect treatment negatively, Angela Joyce (Chapter 3, this volume) adds yet another one; she quickly gets to know about the father's early losses of his parents – whereas *he* clearly says these are bygone things that he does not want to talk about. So, what to do, especially since the therapist sees how the father's failure to mourn these losses affects his relationship with the baby negatively? At first, she 'worked hard with the impact of the rule-bound parents creating a rule-bound baby', such as their obeying the commands from Gina Ford's book. Angela asks what mandate she had to trespass the border at the father's no-go area, 'the locked door at the back of his head', where Andrew had buried his feelings about the early losses. In terms of transference, it was adamantly negative; Andrew feared the therapist's presence, her poking in his pain as it were, and often felt worse than he had before the referral.

If the topic of loss of the parents was necessary to address – for the sake of baby Tommy's well-being – but the father was scared of talking about it and on the verge of leaving treatment, then what to do? Like in Oliver's case above, the baby came to help. Not directly, but in the sense that in one individual session, the father realised that his manner of pushing away his painful mourning – though he did this in an effort to avoid a collapse – might affect Tommy negatively: 'Maybe that's why I do it with Tommy as well . . . pushing him to keep achieving, driving forward, not relaxing'. His concern for the boy's well-being thus helped him diminish obstacles against talking about his childhood pains. His wife also came to help: She told him that Tommy looked for him in the evenings and did not settle easily until seeing Dad. Father concluded that if a six-month-old 'could register and show his feelings about his dad's presence and absence, then in all likelihood a five/six-year-old would certainly have noticed when his dad died and was absent forever'.

In terms of transference I conclude that baby Tommy, or at least the father's concern for him, helped infuse some positive and hopeful notions in this father's initial negative and fearful transference towards Angela. Had Andrew not become a father, he would perhaps never have seen a therapist. Now, he was ushered in by the plights of parenthood plus his affection for the boy. Despite the therapist's disappointment that, after the summer break, 'Andrew's defences were back in place and it proved impossible to re-establish the contact we had had before', some surprising results were obtained, as I mentioned in my general discussion chapter. Here, I have looked at this relative success through another lens, that of the transference, and how the baby acts as co-therapist to encourage the parents to broach hitherto treacherous territories.

Conclusions

This section has neither provided any clear-cut descriptions of how fathers, specifically, manifest transferences in therapy nor any unequivocal recommendations of how to deal with them. This is because, though I think it is highly legitimate to speak of a *father's transference*, I am not prone to use the term *father transference* to *generally* denote what fathers are struggling with. Men become fathers and struggle with being fathers, finding suitable role models, etc. This is true. But to state that men would exhibit 'father transferences' in PIP entails, as I see it, a logical somersault. Transference is a term that refers backwards, to things we experienced previously in life. This is why I labelled the two people speaking about their boss examples of father transferences. I thus referred to the diverging and 'childish' views of their fathers. A man in PIP may experience the therapist similarly, and we might properly call it a father transference. But if so, that term would refer to how he, as a *son*, sees a subjective version of his father in the therapist. I would thus speak of this *father's transference* but not of his *father transference*. To reiterate my point differently, we could speak of a mother's father transference towards her PIP therapist, whatever his/her sex. She thus experiences similarities between the therapist now and her father then.

In my conclusion, I bring out:

- Transference refers to a subjective and unconscious colouring of how the patient experiences the therapist;
- Our understanding of the transference is never 'objective' but is always coloured also by our countertransference;
- Transference appears in individual, family, group, and parent-infant therapy;
- The way we deal with it is not different in principle between these settings;
- The way we deal with it in fathers is similar to how we deal with it in mothers;
- Unique to transferences in PIP is that they occur in a constantly and rapidly changing setting. These vacillations are ushered in not the least by the presence of an immature yet powerful and expressive human being; the baby;
- Another factor, unique to PIP, is that the presence of two or three patients of varying age and maturity paves the way for competitive struggles. A mother may feel the therapist pays too much attention to the baby, or a father may feel pushed aside by the therapist's concern for the mother. If unnoticed, such factors may push transference in a negative direction;
- The important thing is to be aware of, as often and as deeply as possible, the manifestations of transference and countertransference. Whether and when we should address these phenomena explicitly is a decision that the therapist has to ponder on before reaching a decision. One would wish

him/her time and peace of mind to reflect on such issues, but in PIP things often happen on the spot and the therapist needs to improvise. This contributes to the charm and challenges of this kind of work.

ON INTERVENTIONS
TESSA BARADON

In this section I will consider the types of interventions that are portrayed in the chapters. I refer especially to when the author describes what the therapist said and/ or did, and the affective context within which it took place. I have also drawn on their clinical formulations to understand their more conscious intentions, where the therapist was heading in his/her thinking, in saying or doing what s/he did. I would say that an overriding aim in all the interventions was to create triangulation.

To achieve this, perhaps the first intentional activity of the therapist is to create trust that s/he is interested in, and can hold in mind, each of the three members of the family and their togetherness as a unit. This is, in a sense, the work to be done to develop a therapeutic alliance that can be inclusive of the father and help him, mother, and baby tolerate the psychological work of PIP.

The interventions fall within broad groupings:

- Father-focused interventions that address intrapsychic factors that impact the father's capacity to assume his role;
- Mother-focused interventions that attend to mother's mothering issues, as well as to maternal conflicts that compromise the father and his fathering;
- Infant-focused interventions are those that work therapeutically with the baby to enable an experience of 'being known' (Beebe, Lachman, Markese, & Bahrick, 2012a, Beebe et al., 2012b) in his plight of 'fatherlessness';
- Couple-focused interventions to promote co-parenting and, where relevant, reduce conflict;
- Triad-focused interventions, to promote maternal and paternal functioning within the triad.

Father-focused interventions are the most important clinical theme of the book. Fathers' reticence in being a strong paternal presence in their children's lives has been discussed in many chapters. In most of the cases, the therapists could help these men assume effective fathering through interpreting their conflicts around this and giving meaning to their defensive behaviours, for example through understanding their childhood origins. On the one hand, we have Angela Joyce's example in her individual work with Andrew around his bereavements and grieving. He was very ambivalent about opening the 'box at the back of his head', in which unmanageable memories and feelings were deposited. In fact, it was only his wish to be a better father that allowed Joyce an entry, and only a limited one at that. This raises questions, as Joyce suggests, as to what place to give adult material in the therapy?

A vexed issue indeed, when much is unresolved in the adult's mind, and they themselves may be eager for more therapeutic understanding. However, in this case mother and father applied a criteria of 'things were fine now with Tommy'.

Joyce was left with the feeling that this was an interrupted therapy, with her being left with the burden of the unresolved feelings the father could not manage. Yet I think that that permission to address his defences had, from the beginning, been conditional and much was indeed accomplished in terms of the father-baby and triadic relationships, a point that Björn Salomonsson also raises. Perhaps one of the factors differentiating adult psychotherapy and adult-focused work in PIP is that the latter is only part of the PIP therapy, and takes place with the child and family in mind. Before this was offered to Andrew, however, the more characteristic work with the father in the context of the triad occurred. Joyce notes how Rosie was aligned with this: she was keen for Andrew to receive help with this 'no-go' area as it was playing out in their marriage.

Within the broader remit of work with mothers in parent infant psychotherapy, there may be a need to address those aspects of a mother's functioning that compromise the father, especially in his paternal role. For example, much work was done with Celia around her fears of separateness and heightened ambivalence. Her anxieties and conflicts placed Alan in an impossible situation as a father, since any attempts to have a relationship with baby Tommy provoked either rage or depression in Celia. Perez also accounts for the therapeutic interventions she used to address this; interpretation alongside reflection on the predicaments of all three members of the family increased Celia's capacities to mentalize Tommy's need for triadification.

It is not incidental that the parent-focused interventions take place in the presence of their partner and baby. They constitute part of working towards actual triangulation. In this sense, adult/parent-focused interventions in PIP differ from the approaches both in adult psychotherapy and family therapy. In contrast to adult psychotherapy, the direction of travel is not led by free associations but rather by the unfolding developmental agendas of the infant and his parents. In contrast to family therapy, where attention would be on relationships between the parents in the context of the new relationship with the baby, in PIP the therapist's focus is on the (internal) experience of the infant and the parental impact on it. The equal respect and space accorded to the baby as a meaningful actor in the room in itself re-orientates the parents in a way that family therapy would not (personal communication, Minna Daum, 22 April 2018).

Examples of infant-focused interventions differ among the author-therapists in this book, although for all of them the infant is central in their thinking about the therapeutic encounter. The baby informs the therapist about parental projections and other defences and about the relational dynamics in the family and is a patient subject in his own right. Perez addresses baby Oliver directly when she imagines the feelings that underpin his autistic-like withdrawal: 'I leaned over to Oliver and asked him whether he was looking out of the window because he found it so difficult to hear mummy so upset'. This had the effect not only of galvanising his parents into a more mentalising stance but, importantly, of bringing Oliver back into relating.

Jones (Chapter 5) spells out the process of imagining the baby's experience and putting his predicament into words. Her intention is to bring to the mother's awareness her unconscious defensive processes. In the process, she speaks in baby Ben's 'voice': "You've got a belief mummy that I don't want you near me, but actually you can tell just by how I am grabbing you how much I want to be close to you". Thus Jones conveys Ben's message to mother: look and you will see that your transference projections are confounded by my actions. What Ben may gain from this intervention is a validation of his baby needs and intentions, and of his agency. In the face of his mother's incapacity to hear his communications at that point, Jones provides a maternal-therapeutic mind to receive and process his inner world. In my view, this is the critical characteristic of this work.

There is growing sophistication in therapists in empathically imagining the experience of the baby. However, one of the areas of the infant's internal world often less explored by therapists is that of his/her 'father hunger' (Herzog, 2014) in the face of a psychically absent father. This painful hunger is beyond the need for paternal function for development. It touches upon infants' longings and appetites for their fathers. It acknowledges the passion of the infant.

Therapists vary in the interventions they use to address the *couple relationship*. Laznik approaches the couple with a mixture of interpretation and directive explanations. Her use of humour helps her patients to swallow the pill of her authority as the professional third in order to make changes needed by their boy. Emanuel advocates this work to address difficulties in parenting which burden the child. In a well-functioning couple, she suggests, maternal and paternal functions will be embodied in each parent so that the child internalises a parental object with both functions. Emanuel also links the internal parental couple with oedipal issues of exclusion and separateness in young children as they move towards triangulation. She notes the solution reached by her two-year-old patient, Maria, in her preoccupation with circles – 'with no corners to bump against'. I was amused by Louise's countertransference to the princess and Maria's realisation that Louise would not bow to her demands as her parents were prone to do. Accordingly, Louise posed a threat to the status quo.

By *triad-focused interventions* I mean those instances where the therapist moves simultaneously between father, mother and infant in observing, making links and helping to create their triangular space. Such movement took place between Lila and her parents (Chapter 7) when the parents were psychologically able to attend to her communications about feeling lonely and frightened in the face of their withdrawal. The importance of this triadic-focused intervention was that the parents came together and repositioned themselves generationally as the adults who are biologically tasked with protecting their child. For Lila, the recovery of a safe(r) base in the parental couple was critical.

Triadic interventions may also be in action, such as when the therapist rolls a ball to engage the baby in mutual, pleasurable play, which is then handed over to baby and parents. They can be conveyed through gesture, as when the therapist's hand sweeps a circle in the room.

Obviously, some of the variances in the interventions and how they are carried out (beyond the fact that each therapy is co-constructed differently) can be attributed to differences between schools of thought. Much, too, is influenced by local theoretical culture; as Bollas (1996, p. 6) wrote (presumably tongue in cheek) 'Thus the breasts – good and bad – seem to have become the intellectual property of the British to be found in London, while the phallus resides in Paris as the intellectual property of the Lacanians'. The rest must surely be the expression of each therapist's personal idiom.

THE TRIADIC CAPACITY OF THE THERAPIST
KAI VON KLITZING

As outlined in Chapter 2 of this volume, well-balanced and coordinated early triadic experiences (the experience of infants with both mothers and fathers, and with the triadic constellation) are essential for the mentalisation process in early. A well-calibrated alternation between the presence and absence of the nurturing object, as well as between the satisfaction and frustration of needs, is the driving power that leads the child from the pre-concept of an internal object to the representation of the self and the object. The experience of growing up in a triadic relational space (with a mother object, a father object, and possibly many others) seems to be very stimulating. In such constellations the child can experience not only the absence of an important relational object, but also the absence (and presence) of one object in the presence of the third object. We therefore consider it essential to initiate triadic relational processes and to open up triadic spaces for the infant in parent-infant therapy.

In the child, experiencing triadic relationships lays the ground for organising his/her internal world through triangular representations. In this way object representations can become integrated and inclusive. For example, the representation of a mother object includes the image of a third person: a father object. This internal triangulation opens a dynamic capacity in the self of being with an object without becoming a mere narcissistic prolongation of it. This includes the infant accepting that the object is related to other objects as well, which grants autonomy to the infant in a flexible world of relatedness.

The triadic capacity of parents, that is the capacity to be related to one object without excluding the third, helps create a triadic relational space for the baby. For the parents, this is a challenge. In several chapters of this book we have seen how difficult it can be for a mother whose internal world is dominated by dis-integration and projective identification to accept that the baby also has a relationship with the father, without feeling herself to be completely excluded (see case report by Alejandra Perez in Chapter 4 of this volume). Or how a father, whose internal world is dominated either by a complete lack of self-confidence (see case report by Tessa Baradon in Chapter 7 of this volume) or by a tendency towards violent dominance probably driven by his own anxieties (see case report by Amanda Jones in Chapter 5 of this volume) tends to withdraw from the fragile early parent-child relationship.

When we characterise parent-infant therapy as a constant opening of triadic relational processes, it is evident that the therapist needs to have sufficient triadic capacity him/herself. Triadic capacity is needed to be able to enter into intensive contact with both parents and the baby. Even if one parent is physically absent (as in the case report by Amanda Jones) we represent him/her in our minds. To be able to understand what is going on within early relationships we need to be capable of identifying with each protagonist alternately, without forgetting the others (Lebovici, 1983). This requires therapists to be internally flexible, have an advanced resolution of their own triangular conflicts, and be open to dialogue. One has to be in an internal exchange with one's own parental couple, even if one has not experienced one's own parents as a couple, in order to limit one's own phantasies of and desires for exclusive relationships.

We have undergone intensive training in developing and interpreting two-person relationships within the psychoanalytic setting, but we should now focus on improving our triadic capacity. For example, in child analysis we must acknowledge the enormous influence of the real parents on our work with the child. The pioneers of child analyses (such as Hug Helmuth, Anna Freud and Melanie Klein) did not write much about their work with parents, although it is evident that they also saw the parents of the children they treated. In the intensive encounters with young children in analysis, we psychoanalysts are in danger of being led by the phantasy that we ourselves are the better parent for the child. The work of Klitzing (2005), Laplanche (1997), Lebovici (1983), and Novick and Novick (2005) and others has drawn our attention to the need for and benefit of parent work in child analysis. The work with parents challenges us, because it requires us to integrate into our clinical practice not only the relationship with the child, but also with the mother, the father, and the parental couple. In this way we have to move ourselves within several entangled triads as represented in Figure 13.1. Our unconscious is confronted by the primal scene between the real parents, who created the child long before we therapists came into the picture.

Since we psychoanalysts first started to work with babies it was evident that we needed the mothers, because the work done with the baby alone did not make sense. But then came the next challenge: if we could not avoid acknowledging that the baby we saw was borne by the mother in front of us, we could at least imagine that we were replacing an inadequate father. Adopting the position of a good enough father could lead to a better triangulation within the mother-infant relationship. Many fathers supported this attitude if they were not willing to participate in the therapy, had no time when we had time,

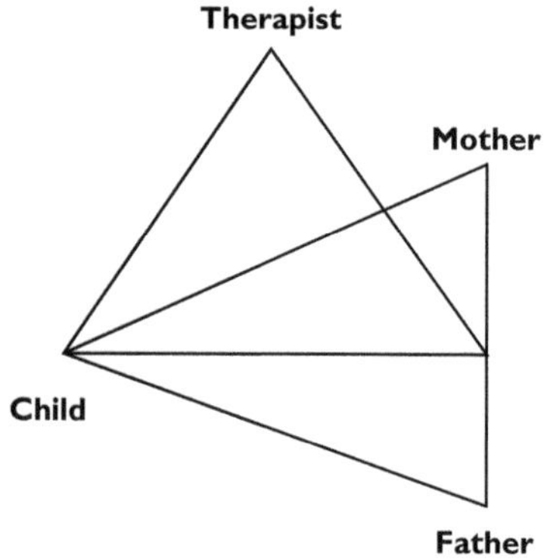

Figure 13.1 Entangled triads in child analytic work.
Source: von Klitzing (2005)

or thought that this kind of talking cure was useless. Or they just felt that we were offering ourselves as the better third so that they saw no place for themselves in the therapeutic endeavour.

The wonderful clinical work presented in this book demonstrates that we are now at the next stage. We acknowledge that the real thirds, the fathers, play an important role in development. We should include them, inviting them to participate and making our work appealing to them. What a challenge for our own triadic capacity! Are we ready to include fathers? Some good examples of inclusive triadic work are reported in this book. We note a lot of detailed technical hints, but also still unsolved problems of triadic work in parent-infant therapies.

Tessa Baradon (Chapter 7, this volume) gives us examples of therapeutic sessions in which she as the therapist actively initiated a movement between a father and his baby in the consulting room. For example, she describes how an immigrant father, full of uncertainty, moved a toy train towards his 8-month-old daughter in order to calm her. In a way, his daughter taught him how fast to move the toy so that she could tolerate his relational approach towards her. He was able to integrate her emotional feedback and the result was that her dysregulated mood was calmed by his approach. The therapist had encouraged careful father-daughter interactional play, which the mother observed sympathetically, leading to an intense triadic experience for all of them.

But of course, as Baradon rightly states, mother-father-baby-therapist can be described as a libidinal constellation which also contains conflicts within itself, especially when sexual rivalry comes into play. The exclamation 'Hey, those [breasts] are mine!' interrupted a deep feeling of identification by a female therapist looking at a baby boy pleasurably handling his mother's breast. Suddenly adult sexual connotations interfered with the seemingly 'innocent' early relationship. What a disruption by the third, the real father! But is the baby not in any case confronted with this kind of confusing message from the sphere of adult sexuality (see Laplanche, 1997)? So the therapist's confusion opens up an opportunity for her to identify with the baby in a disturbing situation, an opportunity she would not have had if she had worked with mother and baby alone.

Alejandra Perez's therapeutic work with a parent-infant constellation in which the mother suffered from borderline problems, and the father did not dare enter into contact with his baby son, shows how helpful it can be to integrate a father into the relational life of a baby (Chapter 4, this volume). Seeing another person be close to her child, the mother became immensely afraid of being completely excluded herself. First, Perez addressed the internal conflictual world of both parents without excluding the other; second, she offered to be a father-like counterpart for both parents, thus providing safety when confronted with anxiety-driven situations; and third, she introduced the voice and view of the father in a way that could be accepted by the mother. She also addressed the baby directly in a way that the father could identify with. The parents were able to identify with Perez's triadic capacity and thus proceed in a triangular way of dealing with triangular aspects of their family relationship.

In her case report, Amanda Jones (Chapter 5, this volume) challenges our claim of integrating fathers into therapy whenever possible. But what should we do if we are told that a specific father is so violent that we fear he could harm the baby and/or his/her mother? This is a critical situation, because we are excluding a meaningful relational partner of the child without really knowing him in person. And we must not forget: we can exclude the father from the consulting room, but we cannot exclude him from the mind of the mother and the growing representational world of the child.

In the case report, mother Anna has moved from one abusive relationship with a male partner to the next, one of whom is now the father of baby boy Ben. And we soon see that there is not only a violent man in reality, but also a violent man in the mind of the mother which she easily projects into the baby: 'Monster boy' she calls her son when she lifts Ben out of his buggy. What a confusion of aggressive and sexual connotations! The unconscious message to Ben is: look, I hate your father because he treated me so violently, but I also sexually desire him, and you have been created by this unresolved mixture of aggression and sexuality. This primary scene leads to the boy being given the incomprehensible but seductive message: the more I hate you, the more I long for you. Many young boys share a bed with their mothers, who tell them that their fathers are bad guys and that their fate is to follow them, first as aggressive and dysregulated little boys, then showing anti-social tendencies during adolescence, and finally ending up as violent men themselves.

So how could we deal with this kind of constellations, when triadic solutions – solutions in which each member of the father-mother-baby triad can integrate his/her ambivalent feelings into him/herself without projecting unaccepted feelings into the other – seem to be out of reach? We cannot wait until the adults have solved their rigid patterns of splitting: they may never reach sufficient integration. Jones does not report what efforts she undertook to meet Ben's father. For the boy it can be of great significance that the therapist has his/her own view of the father, without having looked through the mother's confusing lens. In individual therapy we would not hesitate to deal with the mother's narratives and to acknowledge them as an expression of her psychic reality. But in parent-infant therapy there is also the third, the baby, who needs the therapist's support to develop his/her relational world and his/her internal object representations, which are hopefully not formed solely by the violent and distorted parental partnership.

In her case reports, Marie-Christine Laznik (Chapter 11, this volume) demonstrates her intense efforts to create a space for the paternal function in the parent-infant triad. With a background in Lacanian theory, she has clear concepts of what the paternal function in a family should be: 'I am simply asking you to give the little ship's boy the feeling that there is a captain on board and that if he obeys him, all dangers may be avoided.' Lacan talked about the '*nom du père*' and at the same time of the '*non du père*', which helps the young child to disentangle him/herself from the symbiotic relationship with the mother. But is this really the role of a captain – which implies a quite hierarchical way of solving possible conflicts within the parent-infant triad? In her second case she addresses her perception of collusion between the female therapist and the mother: 'We mothers can feel, we know, and therefore everyone must submit to our knowledge … Then, it's up to us to try and do things differently. But when we are phallic like that, we lose our femininity.' So her recommendation to the mother (with whom she felt very close) is a strategic one: although we know the best for our babies, let the father come into the triadic relationship, let him be part of it, let him execute his paternal function. This will help the baby and make 'us' (mother and female therapist) more desirable and sexually attractive. Laznik recommends supporting the formation of well-balanced triads by assigning each family member his/her place, probably because she holds that a clear hierarchical order is the best means to counter insoluble and dysregulated triangular conflicts.

The aim of this book is to open a creative space for inclusive techniques in parent-child therapy. The chapters and case reports show us, first, that many psychotherapists undertake the adventure of including the father, and second, that their approaches and techniques are highly diverse. So working with fathers in parent-infant therapy is important, but we need far more exchange and discussion between therapists on how technically to handle triadic issues in the therapeutic endeavour.

Chapter 14

And what about mothers?

Tessa Baradon

In this discussion I briefly consider the mothers presented in this book, their prisms of the father as partner and father of their infants, and their impact on the potential for triangulation.

Mothers are present in all the chapters; naturally so, as they are a central part of the fathering equation. We have all concurred with Winnicott, it would appear, that *what mother does* impacts whether and how father and baby get to know each other. Thus, the essence of 'Father' in each family is influenced by both the father's personality, defences, engagement – his personal fathering idiom, and by the mother's emotional and behavioural expressions of her internal representations of him (the 'father in the mother's mind').

It has been noted that the mother may be a facilitator, partner or gatekeeper to the father's relationship with the baby. The mother's representations of the couple dynamics are also critical: is her partner viewed as a man who is potent and desirable, or is he dismissed, devalued? And how does she see herself reflected in the father's eyes, as a woman and as a mother: as an object of desire, contempt, admiration, envy?

Bevington's memoir (Chapter 1) takes the reader through the subtle choreography of his partner in creating a space for the 'otherness' with their new-born. In so doing, we also meet a mother who welcomed her partner/the father into the orbit of 'recognition and familiarity' that had been forming between her and baby since conception. Thus, processes of becoming 'gracefully failing' and good enough parents to an infant become a shared venture. The child, in turn, could engage in a lifelong movement of 'attached' separation.

However, many factors can inhibit or prevent the development of triangulation and co-parenting. Raphael-Leff (Chapter 6) highlights the ecology of relationships – cultural, religious, familial, intrapsychic and interpsychic systems, within which orientations to fathering develop. The same, of course, applies to mothers. When von Klitzing (Chapter 2) discusses the role of the father in relation to the child's hatred of the mother, I understand that he is referring to triadic management of ambivalence. Some measure of ambivalence is part and parcel of familial life. For the mother it includes her own ambivalence toward her child, the child's toward her, and – as we see in the contributions to this book – in the father towards both.

The clinical chapters describe aspects of maternal ambivalence towards the father. Different maternal profiles are considered. On the one hand are those mothers who seem to maintain a basic capacity to mentalise about their partner even while struggling deeply with their own anxieties. In the family presented by Angela Joyce (Chapter 3), the mother – Rosie – was beset by feelings of failure and helplessness following a traumatic birth and screaming baby. Joyce described a process of splitting in the couple wherein mother projected her self-condemnation onto her partner and was then critical of her his perceived incompetence. The therapy appeared to quite quickly resolve the tension between mother's disappointment in him and her wishes for intimacy with him and for greater engagement with their son. Similarly, Anna and Sade, the mothers introduced in Segal's and Fagin's first cases (Chapters 8 and 9), maintained some awareness of the difficulties their partners faced and the impact of their states of mind on their capacities as spouse and father. A central trigger to recovery in these mothers was the concern for the well-being of the infant, and the recognition of a role for the father in this. Thus, it seems that *a capacity for sustained mentalisation and an internal representation of a functioning triad are key to a mother's inclusiveness of father in a therapeutic process*. Perhaps it is the capacity to mentalise that underpins the wish to re-find intimacy with her partner (as known before pregnancy and birth), which facilitates the work with ambivalence. While this may not be conscious at the time of referral, the therapy can become a space for desire to emerge.

Laznik (Chapter 11) presents another viewpoint. She suggests that for triadification to occur, the mother must forgo her omnipotent phantasy that 'she knows best'. She directly addresses the phallic mother who asserts possession of both feminine and masculine, maternal and paternal attributes, and leaves no room for the man in her bed or as a 'real father' 'worthy of his name'. Failure of *nom du père* in both the families she is discussing resulted in the child facing psychic catastrophe: maternal engulfment. I believe that the rapid transformation of the families into functioning triads through therapy derived from latent healthy premises in both parents and child. Key to this was the mother's buried representation of a potent man/lover; as Laznik writes re the first case: 'The mother in a sense indicated to her son that there was indeed a phallus beyond himself'. This knowledge in mother was complemented by her child's extraordinary capacity to communicate his predicament in his play, and by father's capacity to distinguish, with the help of the analyst, between a 'captain of the ship' and a 'screaming sergeant'.

By contrast, the chapters by Perez (Chapter 4) and Jones (Chapter 5) present mothers in whom a dyadic configuration is compelling and exclusive of a third. In this mental configuration there is no capacity to consider the experience of either the object of enmeshment or of exclusion. For Celia (Chapter 3) a merged fusion with her baby was a defence against psychic collapse. This omnipotent phantasy, which is devouring for the child, was slowly reigned in through the therapeutic work. In the therapeutic encounter there was place for each individual in the family, and through this triangulation could also take root. The infant's autistic-like carapace was relinquished in favour of lively engagement.

An even more stark reality confronted Anna, with whom Jones (Chapter 5) engaged in therapeutic work to protect her and her baby from her compulsion to repeat deeply damaging internal scenarios in her relationship with her partner and with her baby. In a sense, Jones's chapter addresses a perverse version of the motherhood constellation, wherein an abusive internal mother is re-embodied in a violent and abusive man, father of her baby. Aptly, Jones describes the mother's illness as of 'transgenerational relational origin'. In her illness, Anna had lost sight of her baby *qua* baby; he was a dangerous 'monster boy ... monster man'. Through the relationship with Jones and the therapeutic work, Anna started to build a different internal scenario, one of a 'new concerned couple who care about both her and the development of her baby'. This experience was transformational in that it kindled more positive representations of both her mothering and femininity, and freed her baby from his entrapment in his mother's hostile projections.

In sum

What is reconfirmed for me in the process of writing this discussion is that a book about fathers is necessarily also about the mothers of their children, and any observation of the baby must include both his parents. Unfortunately for children, this is not yet common practice in either therapy or even in the courts.

Bibliography

Abelin, E. (1971). The role of the father in the separation – Individuation process. In J. McDevitt & C. Settlage (eds.), *Separation – Individuation* 229–52. New York: International Universities Press.

Abelin, E. L. (1975). Some further observations and comments on the earliest role of the father. *International Journal of Psychoanalysis*, 56, 293–302.

Abraham, E., Hendler, T., Shapira-Lichter, I., Kanat-Maymon, K., Zagoory-Sharon, O., & Feldman, R. (2014a). Brain basis of human fatherhood. *Proceedings of the National Academy of Sciences*, July, 111(27), 9792–97. DOI: 10.1073/pnas.1402569111.

Abraham, E., Hendler, T., Shapira-Lichter, I., Kanat-Maymon, Y., Zagoory-Sharon, O., & Feldman, R. (2014b). Father's brain is sensitive to childcare experiences. *Psychological and Cognitive Sciences*, 27, 9792–97.

Addis, M. E., & Mahalik, J. R. (2003). Men, masculinity, and the contexts of help seeking. *American Psychologist*, 58(1), 5–14. DOI: 10.1037/0003-066X.58.1.5.

Allison, E., & Fonagy, P. (2016). When is truth relevant? *The Psychoanalytic Quarterly*, 85(2), 275–303.

Atzil, S., Hendler, T., Zagoory-Sharon, O., Winetraub, Y., & Feldman, R. (2012). Synchrony and specificity in the maternal and the paternal brain: Relations to oxytocin and vasopressin. *Journal of the American Academy of Child and Adolescent Psychiatry*, 51(8), 798–811.

Balint, M. (1949). Early developmental states of the ego. Primary object love. *International Journal of Psychoanalysis*, 30, 265–73.

Baradon, T. (2010). *Relational Trauma in Infancy: Psychoanalytic, Attachment and Neuropsychological Contributions to Parent-Infant Psychotherapy.* London: Routledge.

Baradon, T. (2016). The clinical framework and participants. In T. Baradon with M. Biseo, C. Broughton, J. James, & A. Joyce (eds.), *The Practice of Psycho-Analytic Parent-Infant Psychotherapy: Claiming the Baby.* 2nd Edition, 30–40. London, New York: Routledge.

Baradon, T., Salomonsson, B., & von Klitzing, K. (2014). Diskussion – Wer ist der patient in der Eltern-Kleinkind-Therapie? (Discussion: Who is the patient in parent-infant therapy?). *Kinderanalyse*, 22(1), 71–87.

Barrows, P. (1999). Fathers in parent-infant psychotherapy. *Journal of Infant Mental Health*, 20(3), 333–45.

Barrows, P. (2004). Fathers and families: Locating the ghost in the nursery. *Journal of Infant Mental Health*, 25, 408–23.

Bateman, A. W. (1998). Thick- and thin-skinned organisations and enactment in borderline and narcissistic disorders. *The International Journal of Psychoanalysis*, 79, 13–25.
Beebe, B., Lachman, F., Markese, S., & Bahrick, L. (2012a). On the origins of disorganized attachment and internal working models: Paper l: A dyadic systems approach. *Psychoanalytic Dialogues*, 22, 253–72.
Beebe, B., Lachman, F., Markese, S., Buck, K. A., Bahrick, L., & Chen, H. (2012b). On the origins of disorganized attachment and internal working models: Paper II: A dyadic systems approach. *Psychoanalytic Dialogues*, 22(3), 352–74.
Belsky, J., & Volling, B. L. (1987). Exploring family system processes. In P. W. Berman & F. A. Pederson (eds.), *Men's Transition to Parenthood: Longitudinal Studies of Early Family Experience* 3–65. New Jersey: LEA.
Belsky, J., Youngblade, L., Rovine, M., & Volling, B. (1991). Patterns of marital change and parent-child interaction. *Journal of Marriage and Family*, 53, 487–98.
Bergbom, I., Modh, C., Lundgren, I., & Lindwall, L. (2016). First-time pregnant women's experiences of their body in early pregnancy. *Scandinavian Journal of Caring Sciences*. DOI: 10.1111/scs.12372.
Bion, W. (1962). *Learning from Experience*. London: Tavistock Publications.
Bion, W. R. (1990). *Brazilian Lectures*. London: Karnac Books.
Biseo, M. (2016). Parent infant psychotherapy: Engaging and beginning the work. In T. Baradon with M. Biseo, C. Broughton, J. James, & A. Joyce (eds.), *The Practice of Psycho-Analytic Parent-Infant Psychotherapy: Claiming the Baby*. 2nd Edition. London, New York: Routledge.
Blos, P. (1987). Freud and the father complex. *Psychoanalytic Study of the Child*, 42, 425–41.
Bollas, C. (1979). The transformational object. *International Journal of Psychoanalysis*, 60(1), 97–107.
Bollas, C. (1996). Figures and their functions: On the oedipal structure of psychoanalysis. *Psychoanalytic Quarterly*, LXV, 1–20.
Bollas, C. (2013). *Catch Them before They Fall*. London: Routledge.
Borens, R. (1993). Vater sein dagegen sehr. *Zs.psa.Theorie u.Praxis*, 8, 19–31.
Bouchard, S., Sabourin, S., Lussier, Y., & Villeneuve, E. (2009). Relationship quality and stability in couples where one partner suffers from Borderline Personality Disorder. *Journal of Marital and Family Therapy*, 35(4), 446–55.
Bowen, M. (1978). *Family Therapy in Clinical Practice*. New York: Aronson.
Bretherton, I. (2010). Fathers in attachment theory and research: A review. *Early Child Development and Care*, 180, 9–23. DOI: 10.1080/03004430903414661.
Britton, R. (1989). The missing link: Parental sexuality in the Oedipus complex. In R. Britton, M. Feldman, & E. O'Shaugnessy (eds.), *The Oedipus Complex Today: Clinical Implications* 83–101. London: Karnac Books.
Britton, R. (2004). Subjectivity, objectivity, and triangular space. *Psychoanalytic Quarterly*, 73, 47–61.
Brizendine, L. (2010). *The Male Brain*. New York: Books.
Burgess, A. (1997). *Fatherhood Reclaimed: The Making of the Modern Father*. London: Vermillion, Random House.
Burlingham, D. (1943). In the first discussion of scientific controversies: On Mrs Susan Isaacs' paper 'The nature and function of phantasy'. In P. King & R. Steiner (eds.), *The Freud–Klein Controversies 1941–1945* 322–56. London: Routledge, 1991.

Carneiro, C., Corboz-Warnery, A., & Fivaz-Depeursinge, E. (2006). The prenatal Lausanne Trilogue play: A new observational assessment tool of the prenatal co-parenting alliance. *Infant Mental Health Journal*, 27(2), 207–28.

Corboz, A., Forni, P., & Fivaz, E. (1989). Le jeu à trois entre père, mère et bébé: Une méthode d'analyse des interactions visuelles triadiques. *Neuropsychiatrie De L'enfance*, 37(1), 23–33.

Corboz Warnery, A., Fivaz Depeursinge, E., Bettens, C. G., & Favez, N. (1993). Systemic analysis of father-mother-baby interactions: The Lausanne triadic play. *Infant Mental Health Journal*, 14(4), 298–316.

Cowan, C. P. (1996). Becoming parents: What has to change for couples? In C. Clulow (ed.), *Partners Becoming Parents*. London: Sheldon Press.

Cowan, P. A., & Cowan, C. P. (1987). Men's involvement in parenthood: Identifying the antecedents and understanding the barriers. In P. W. Berman & F. A. Pederson (eds.), *Men's Transitions into Parenthood: Longitudinal Studies of Early Family Experience* 145–74. Hillsdale, NJ: LEA.

Davids, M. F. (2002). Fathers in the internal world: From boy to man to father. In S. Budd, J. Trowell, & A. Etchegoyen (Vol. eds.), New library of psychoanalysis. *The Importance of Fathers – A Psychoanalytic Re-Evaluation*. Hove: Brunner-Routledge.

Davies, N., & Eagle, G. (2013). Conceptualizing the paternal function: Maleness, masculinity, or thirdness? *Contemporary Psychoanalysis*, 49(4), 559–85.

De Montigny-Malenfant, B., Santerre, M.-E., Bouchard, S., Sabourin, S., Lazarides, A., & Belanger, C. (2013). Couples' negative interaction behaviors and Borderline Personality Disorder. *The American Journal of Family Therapy*, 41(3), 259–71.

Diamond, M. J. (2017). Recovering the father in mind and flesh: History, triadic functioning, and developmental implications. *Psychoanalytic Quarterly*, 86(2), 297–334.

Dugmore, N. (2014). Flexing the frame: contemplating the use of multiple ports of entry in parent–infant psychotherapy. *Infant Mental Health Journal*, 35, 366–375.

Eizirik, C. L. (2015). The father, the father function, the father principle: Some contemporary psychoanalytic developments. *The Psychoanalytic Quarterly*, 84(2), 335–50.

Emde, R. N. (1988). Development terminable and interminable. I. Innate and motivational factors from infancy. *International Journal of Psychoanalysis*, 69(1), 23–42.

Etchegoyen, A. (2002). Psychoanalytic ideas about fathers. In S. Budd (Series ed.) & J. Trowell, & A. Etchegoyen (Vol. eds.), New library of psychoanalysis. *The Importance of Fathers – A Psychoanalytic Re-Evaluation* 20–42. Hove: Brunner-Routledge.

Faimberg, H. (1988). The telescoping of generations: Genealogy of certain identifications. *Contemporary Psychoanalysis*, 24, 99–117.

Favez, N., Lopes, F., Bernard, M., Frascarolo, F., Lavanchy Scaiola, C., Corboz-Warnery, A., et al. (2012). The development of family alliance from pregnancy to toddlerhood and child outcomes at five years. *Family Process*, 51(4), 542–56.

Feldman, R. (2003). Infant-mother and infant-father synchrony: The coregulation of positive arousal. *Infant Mental Health Journal*, 24(1), 1–23.

Ferenczi, S. (1933). Confusion of tongues between adult and the child. In In M. Balint (ed.), *Final Contributions to the Problems and Methods of Psychoanalysis* (1955) 156–67. London: Maresfield.

Field, T. (1978). Interactions behaviour of primary versus secondary caretaker fathers. *Developmental Psychology*, 14, 83–184.

Field, T. (1998). Maternal depression effects on infants and early interventions. *Preventive Medicine*, 27(2), 200–03.

Fitzgerald, H. E., Bocknek, E. L., Hossain, H., & Roggman, L. (2015). Reflections on fathers and infant mental health. *Infant Mental Health Journal*, 36(1), 75–77.

Fivaz-Depeursinge, E., Cairo, S., Scaiola, C. L., & Favez, N. (2012). Nine month-olds' triangular interactive strategies with their parents' couple in low-coordination families: A descriptive study. *Infant Mental Health Journal*, 33(1), 10–21.

Fivaz-Depeursinge, E., & Corboz-Warnery, A. (1999). *The Primary Triangle: A Developmental Systems View of Mothers, Fathers, and Infants*. New York: Basic Books.

Fivaz-Depeursinge, E., & Corboz-Warnery, A. (2000). Prenatal co-parenting alliance and infant's handling of triangular interaction at 4 months. *Infant Mental Health Journal*, 21(4–5), 373.

Fonagy, P., Luyten, P., Allison, E., & Campbell, C. (2017). What we have changed our minds about: Part 2. Borderline Personality Disorder, epistemic trust and developmental significance of social communication. *Borderline Personality Disorder and Emotion Dysregulation*, 4, Article 9. DOI: 10.1186/s40479-017-0062-8.

Fonagy, P., & Target, M. (1995). Understanding the violent patient: The use of the body and the role of the father. *The International Journal of Psychoanalysis*, 76, 487–501.

Fonagy, P., & Target, M. (2000a). Playing with reality: III. The persistence of dual psychic reality in borderline patients. *The International Journal of Psychoanalysis*, 81(5), 853–73.

Fonagy, P., & Target, M. (2000b). Mentalisation and the changing aims of child psychoanalysis. In K. von Klitzing, P. Tyson, & D. Bürgin (eds.), *Psychoanalysis in Childhood and Adolescence* 129–39. Basel: Karger.

Fonagy, P., & Target, M. (2005). Bridging the transmission gap: An end to an important mystery of attachment research? *Attachment & Human Development*, 7(3), 333–43.

Ford, G. (2006). *The New Contented Little Baby Book*. London: Vermillion.

Fraiberg, S. (1987). *Selected Writings of Selma Fraiberg*. Columbus, OH: Ohio State University Press.

Freeman, T. (2008). Psychoanalytic concepts of fatherhood: Patriarchal paradoxes and the presence of an absent authority. *Studies in Gender and Sexuality*, 9(2), 113–39.

Freud, A. (1943). Contribution to the discussion of Susan Isaac's paper. In P. King & R. Steiner (eds.), *The Freud–Klein Controversies 1941–1945* 415–25. London: Routledge, 1991.

Freud, H. C. (2011). *Electra vs. Oedipus: The Drama of the Mother-Daughter Relationship*. London: Routledge.

Freud, S. (1895). *Project for a Scientific Psychology*. Standard Edition 1, 281–391. London: Hogarth Press.

Freud, S. (1905). *Three Essays on the Theory of Sexuality*. Standard Edition 7, 125–243. London: Hogarth Press.

Freud, S. (1909a). *Analyse der Phobie eines fünfjährigen Knaben ('Der Kleine Hans')*. GW, Vol. 7, 243–377.

Freud, S. (1909b). *Analysis of a Phobia in a Five-Year-Old Boy*. Standard Edition 10, 1–150. London: Hogarth Press.

Freud, S. (1909c). *Family Romances*. Standard Edition 9, 235–42.

Freud, S. (1912). *On the Universal Tendency to Debasement in the Sphere of Love (Contributions to the Psychology of Love II)*. Standard Edition 11, 177–90. London: Hogarth Press.

Freud, S. (1913). *Totem and Taboo*. Standard Edition 8, vii–162. London: Hogarth Press.

Freud, S. (1914a). *Mourning and Melancholia*. Standard Edition 14, 237–58. London: Hogarth Press.

Freud, S. (1914b). *Remembering, Repeating and Working Through*. Standard Edition 12, 255–69. London: Hogarth Press.

Freud, S. (1914c). *On Narcissism: An Introduction*. Standard Edition 14, 67–102. London: Hogarth Press.

Freud, S. (1921). *Group Psychology and the Analysis of the Ego*. Standard Edition 18, 65–144. London: Hogarth Press.

Freud, S. (1925–6). *Inhibitions, Symptoms and Anxiety*. Standard Edition 20, 87–178. London: Hogarth Press.

Freud, S. (1926a). *Inhibitions, Symptoms and Anxiety*. Standard Edition 20, 25–176. London: Hogarth Press.

Freud, S. (1926b). *The Question of Lay Analysis*. Standard Edition 20, 177–258. London: Hogarth Press.

Freud, S. (1927). *The Future of an Illusion*. Standard Edition 21, 1–56. London: Hogarth Press.

Freud, S. (1930a). *Civilization and Its Discontents*. Standard Edition 21, 57–146. London: Hogarth Press.

Freud, S. (1930b). Das Unbehagen in der Kultur. GW 14, S. 419.

Freud, S. (1937). *Analysis Terminable and Interminable*. Standard Edition 23, 211–53. London: Hogarth Press.

Freud, S. (1939). *Moses and Monotheism*. Standard Edition 23, 1–138. London: Hogarth Press.

Freud, S. (1950). *Project for a Scientific Psychology* (1950 [1895]). Standard Edition 1, 281–391. London: Hogarth Press.

Frosh, S. (1997). Fathers' ambivalence (too). In W. Hollway & B. Featherstone (eds.), *Mothering and Ambivalence* 37–53. London and New York: Routledge.

Furman, E. (1974). *A Child's Parent Dies: Studies in Childhood Bereavement*. New Haven, CT: Yale University Press.

Galdiolo, S., & Roskan, I. (2016). From me to us: The construction of family alliance. *Journal of Infant Mental Health*, 37(1), 29–44.

Genesoni, L., & Tallandini, M. A. (2009). Men's psychological transition to fatherhood: An analysis of the literature, 1989–2008. *Birth. Issues in Perinatal Care*, 36(4), 305–18.

George, C., Kaplan, N., & Main, M. (1985). *Adult Attachment Interview Protocol*. 2nd Edition. Unpublished manuscript. Berkeley, CA: University of California at Berkeley.

Gergely, G., Egyed, K., & Kiraly, I. (2007). On pedagogy. *Developmental Science*, 10(1), 139–46.

Glasser, M. (1985). The 'weak spot' – Some observations on male sexuality. *International Journal of Psychoanalysis*, 66, 405–14.

Golombok, S. (2017). Parenting in new family forms current opinion. *Psychology*, 15, 76–80.

Goodman, S. H., Lusby, C. M., Thompson, K., Newport, D. J., & Stowe, Z. N. (2014). Maternal depression in association with fathers' involvement with their infants: Spillover or compensation/buffering? *Infant Mental Health Journal*, 35(5), 495–508.

Gordon, I., & Feldman, R. (2008). Synchrony in the triad: A microlevel process model of coparenting and parent-child interactions. *Family Process*, 47(4), 465–79.

Gorell Barnes, G. (2017). *Staying Attached: Fathers and Children in Troubled Times*. London: Karnac.

Green, A. (2004). Thirdness and psychoanalytic concepts. *The Psychoanalytic Quarterly*, 73(1), 99–135.

Greenacre, P. (1957). The childhood of the artist-libidinal phase development and giftedness. *Psychoanalytic Study of the Child*, 12, 47–72.

Gurwitt, A. (1976). Aspects of prospective fatherhood – A case report. *Psychoanalytic Study of the Child*, 31, 237–71.

Gutierrez-Galve, L., Stein, A., Hanington, L., Heron, J., & Ramchandani, P. (2015). Paternal depression in the postnatal period and child development: Mediators and moderators. *Pediatrics*, 135(2), e339–47.

Herbert, J., & Fine, C. (2017). Is testosterone the key to sex differences in human behaviour? *The Psychologist*, 30, 44–49.

Herzog, J. (1982). Patterns of expectant fatherhood: A study of the fathers of a group of premature infants. In S. Cath, A. Gurwitt, & J. M. Ross (eds.), *Father and Child – Developmental and Clinical Perspectives* 301–14. Boston, MA: Little, Brown & Co.

Herzog, J. (1998). Frühe Interaktion und Repräsentanzen: Die Rolle des Vaters in frühen und späten Triaden; der Vater als Förderer der Entwicklung von der Dyade zur Triade. In D. Bürgin (ed.), *Triangulierung* 162–78. Stuttgart: Schattauer.

Herzog, J. M. (1980). Sleep disturbance and father hunger in 18- to 28-month-old boys. *Psychoanalytic Study of the Child*, 45, 219–33.

Herzog, J. M. (1988). Preodipal Oedipus: The father-child dialogue. In G. H. Pollock & J. M. Ross (eds.), *Oedipus Papers* 475–91. Madison, CT: International Universities Press.

Herzog, J. M. (2014). *Father Hunger: Explorations with Adults and Children*. New York: Routledge.

Holmberg, J. R., & Olds, D. (2014). Father attendance in nurse home visitation. *Infant Mental Health Journal*, 36(1), 127–39.

Holmes, E. K., Cowan, P. C., Cowan, C. P., & Hawkins, A. (2013). Marriage, fatherhood, and parenting programming. In N. J. Cabrera & C. S. Tamis-LeMonda (eds.), *Handbook of Father Involvement: Multidisciplinary Perspectives*. 2nd Edition, 438–54. New York: Routledge.

Hopkins, J. (1994). Therapeutic interventions in infancy. Crying babies: Who is crying about what? First published in *Psychoanalytic Psychotherapy* 8, 141–52 (1994) and amended for J. Raphael-Leff (ed.) (2003). *Parent-Infant Psychodynamics: Wild Things, Mirrors and Ghosts*. London: Whurr. Republished in an Independent Mind: Collected papers of Juliet Hopkins Edited by Ann Horne and Monica Lanyado (2015) London: Routledge.

Hossain, Z., Field, T., Gonzalez, J., Malphurs, J., & Del Valle, C. (1994). Infants of 'depressed' mothers interact better with their nondepressed fathers. *Infant Mental Health Journal*, 15, 348–57.

Hrdy, S. B. (2016). Development plus social selection in the evolution of 'emotionally modern' humans. In C. L. Meehan & A. N. Crittenden (eds.), *Childhood: Origins, Evolution and Implications* 11–44. Albuquerque, NM: University of New Mexico Press.

ICD-10. *The International Classification of Diseases Version 10*. Hyattsville, MD: The National Center for Health Statistics (NCHS).

IPA Debates. 2014. Retrieved from http://www.ipa.org.uk/en/Debates/Paternal_Function.aspx.

Jones, A. (2006a). How video can bring to view pathological defensive processes and facilitate the creation of triangular space in perinatal parent-infant psychotherapy. *Infant Observation*, 9(2), 109–23.

Jones, A. (2006b). Levels of change in parent-infant psychotherapy. *The Journal of Child Psychotherapy*, 32(3), 295–311.

Joseph, B. (1985). Transference: The total situation. *International Journal of Psychoanalysis*, 66, 447–454.

Kernberg, O. (1999). Plädoyer für eine 'Drei-Personen-Psychologie'. *Psyche*, 53(9/10), 878–93.

Kim, P., Leckman, J. F., Mayes, L. C., Feldman, R., Wang, X., & Swain, J. E. (2010). The plasticity of human maternal brain: Longitudinal changes in brain anatomy during the early postpartum period. *Behavioral Neuroscience*, 124(5), 695–700.

Kim, P., Rigo, P., Mayes, L. C., Feldman, R., Leckman, J. F., & Swain, J. E. (2014). Neural plasticity in fathers of human infants. *Social Neuroscience*, 9(5), 522–35.

Klein, M. (1928). Early stages of Oedipus conflict. *International Journal of Psychoanalysis*, 9, 167–80.

Klein, M. (1952). The origins of transference. In R. Money-Kyrle (ed.), *Envy and Gratitude and Other Works* (1980 ed., vol. 3, pp. 48–56). London: Hogarth Press.

Klitzing, K. v. (2005). Rivalen oder Bündnispartner? Die Rolle der Eltern bei der analytischen Arbeit mit Kindern. *Kinderanalyse*, 13(2), 113–122.

Klitzing, K. v., & Bürgin, D. (2005). Parental capacities for triadic relationships during pregnancy: Early predictors of children's behavioral and representational functioning at preschool age. *Infant Mental Health Journal*, 26(1), 19–39.

Klitzing, K. v., Simoni, H., Amsler, F., & Bürgin, D. (1999). The role of the father in early family interactions. *Infant Mental Health Journal*, 20(3), 222–37.

Klitzing, K. v., Simoni, H., & Bürgin, D. (1999). Infant development and early triadic family relationships. *Journal of Psychoanalysis*, 80, 71–89.

Klitzing, K. v., & Stadelmann, S. (2011). Das Kind in der triadischen Beziehungswelt. *Psyche-Zeitschrift für Psychoanalyse und Ihre Anwendungen*, 65(9–10), 953–72. Retrieved from http://gateway.isiknowledge.com/gateway/Gateway.cgi?GWVersion=2&SrcAuth=ResearchSoft&SrcApp=EndNote&DestLinkType=FullRecord&DestApp=WOS&KeyUT=000294653400007.

Kramer, S., & Prall, R. (1978). The role of the father in the preoedipal years. *Journal American Psychoanalytic Association*, 26, 143–61.

Lacan, J. (1953). Funktion und Feld des Sprechens und der Sprache in der Psychoananlyse. In J. Lacan (ed.), *Schriften*. 1st Edition, 71–169. Olten: Walter.

Lacan, J. (1998a). *Le Séminaire, Livre IV: La Relation d'objet*. Paris: Seuil.

Lacan, J. (1998b). La forclusion du Nom-du-Père (The foreclosure of the name of the father). In J.-A. Miller (ed.), *Le séminaire vol. 5. Les formations de l'inconscient (The Seminar, Vol. 5. Formations of the Unconscious)* 143–59. Paris: Editions du Seuil.

Lacan, J. (2005). Aggressiveness in psychoanalysis (1948). In his *Écrits*. Translated by Bruce Fink. New York: Norton.

Lacan, J. (2017). *The Seminar of Jacques Lacan, Book V: Formations of the Unconscious*. Cambridge: Polity Press.

Lamb, M. E. (1975). Fathers. *Human Development*, 18, 245–66.

Lamb, M. E. (ed.). (1976). *The Role of the Father in Child Development.* New York: Wiley.
Lamb, M. E. (1977a). Father-infant and mother-infant interaction in the first year of life. *Child Development*, 48, 167–81.
Lamb, M. E. (1977b). The development of mother-infant and father-infant attachments in the second year of life. *Developmental Psychology*, 13(6), 637–48. DOI: 10.1037/0012-1649.13.6.637.
Lamb, M. E. (2002). Infant-father attachments and their impact on child development. In C. Tamis-LeMonda & N. Cabrera (eds.), *Handbook of Father-Involvement* 93–117. Hillsdale, NJ: Erlbaum.
Laplanche, J. (1997). The theory of seduction and the problem of the other. *The International Journal of Psycho-analysis*, 78 (Pt 4), 653–666.
Laplanche, J. (2002). Sexuality and attachment in metapsychology. In D. Widlöcher (ed.), *Infantile Sexuality and Attachment* 37–63. New York: Other Press.
Laplanche, J., & Pontalis, J. B. (1973). *The Language of Psychoanalysis.* London: Hogarth Press.
Laslett, P. (1983). *The World We Have Lost: Further Explored.* London: Routledge.
Layland, W. R. (1981). In search of a loving father. *International Journal of Psychoanalysis*, 62, 215–24.
Laznik, M. C. (2009). The Lacanian theory of the drive: An examination of possible gains for research on autism. *The Journal of the Centre for Freudian Analysis and Research*, 19, 41–62.
Laznik, M. C. (2014). Empathie émotionnelle et autisme. In M. D. Amy (ed.), *Psychanalyse et autismes: évolution des pratiques, recherches et articulations.* Toulouse: Erès.
Lebovici, S. (1983). *Le nourrison, la mère et le psychanalyste.* Paris: Édition du Centurion.
Levine, H., Jørgensen, N., Martino-Andrade, A., Mendiola, J., Weksler-Derri, D., Mindlis, I., et al. (2017). Temporal trends in sperm count: A systematic review and meta-regression analysis. *Human Reproduction (Update)*, 23, 646–59.
Lewis, C. (1986). *Becoming a Father.* Milton Keynes: Open University Press.
Liebman, S. J., & Abell, S. C. (2000). The forgotten parent no more: A psychoanalytic reconsideration of fatherhood. *Psychoanalytic Psychology*, 17(1), 88–105.
Lyons-Ruth, K. (1998). Implicit relational knowing: It's role in development and psychoanalytic treatment. *Infant Mental Health Journal*, 19, 282–89.
Lyons-Ruth, K., Yellin, C., Melnick, S., & Attwood, G. (2003). Childhood experiences of trauma and loss have different relations to maternal unresolved and helpless states of mind on the AAI. *Attachment & Human Development*, 5(4), 330–52.
Mahler, M., & Gosliner, B. (1955). On symbiotic child psychosis: Genetic, dynamic and restitutive aspects. *Psychoanalytic Study of the Child*, 10, 195–212.
Maiello, S. (2007). Containment and differentiation: Notes on the observer's maternal and paternal function. *Infant Observation*, 10(1), 41–49.
Main, M., & Hesse, E. (1990). Parents' unresolved traumatic experiences are related to infant disorganized attachment status: Is frightened and/or frightening parental behavior the linking mechanism. In M. Greenberg, D. Cicchetti, & E. M. Cummings (eds.), Foundation series on mental health and development. *Attachment in the Preschool Years: Theory, Research, and Intervention* 161–84. Chicago, IL: University of Chicago Press.

Mann, D. (1999). *Erotic Transference and Countertransference: Clinical Practice in Psychotherapy*. London: Routledge.

Marks, M. (2002). Letting fathers in. In J. Trowell & A. Etchegoyen (eds.), *The Importance of Fathers: A Psychoanalytic Re-Evaluation* 93–106. East Sussex: Brunner-Routledge.

Marks, M., & Lovestone, S. (1995). The role of the father in parental postnatal mental health. *The British Journal of Medical Psychology*, 68(2), 157–68.

May, U. (2001). Abraham's discovery of the 'bad mother': A contribution to the history of the theory of depression. *International Journal of Psychoanalysis*, 82, 283–305.

McDougal, J. (1993). The dead father: On early psychic trauma and its relation to disturbance in sexual identity and to creative activity. In D. Breen (ed.), *The Gender Conundrum: Contemporary Psychoanalytic Perspectives on Femininity and Masculinity* 233–57. London: Routledge.

McDougall, J. (1986). Parent loss. In A. Rothstein (ed.), *The Reconstruction of Trauma* 135–52. Madison, WI: International Universities Press.

McHale, J., Fivaz-Depeursinge, E., Dickstein, S., Robertson, J., & Daley, M. (2008). New evidence for the social embeddedness of infants' early triangular capacities. *Family Process*, 47(4), 445–63.

McHale, J., & Phares, V. (2015). From dyads to family systems: A bold new direction for infant mental health practice. *Zero to Three Journal*, 35, 1–8.

McHale, J., Talbot, J., & Baker, J. (2009). Sharing the love: Prebirth adult attachment status and coparenting adjustment during early infancy. *Parenting: Science and Practice*, 9(1–2), 56–77.

McWilliams, N. (2011). *Understanding Personality Structure in the Clinical Process: Psychoanalytic Diagnosis*. 2nd Edition. New York: The Guilford Press.

Mead, M. (1957). Changing patterns of parent-child relations in an urban culture. *International Journal of Psychoanalysis*, 38, 369–78.

Melman, C. (2005). *L'homme sans gravité: jouir à tout prix*. Paris: Gallimard.

Mészáros, J. (2010). Building blocks toward contemporary trauma theory: Ferenczi's paradigm shift. *American Journal of Psychoanalysis*, 70(4), 328–40.

Miano, A., Grosselli, L., Roepke, S., & Dziobek, I. (2017). Emotional dysregulation in Borderline Personality Disorder and its influence on communication behavior and feelings in romantic relationships. *Behaviour Research and Therapy*, 95, 148–57.

Morgan, M. (2001). First contacts – The therapist's 'couple state of mind' as a factor in the containment of couples seen for consultation. In F. Grier (ed.), *Brief Encounters with Couples – Some Analytic Perspectives*. London: Karnac Books.

Nelson, S. K., Kushlev, K., English, T., Dunn, E. W., & Lyubomirsky, S. (2013). In defense of parenthood: Children are associated with more joy than misery. *Psychological Science*, 24, 3–10.

Novick, K. K., & Novick, J. (2005). *Working with Parents Makes Therapy Work*. Lanham: Jason Aronson.

Olliac, B., Crespin, G., Laznik, M.-C., Cherif Idrissi El Ganouni, O., Sarradet, J.-L., Bauby, C., et al. (2017). Infant and dyadic assessment in early community-based screening for autism spectrum disorder with the PREAUT grid. *PLoS One*, 12(12), e0188831.

Palacio Espasa, F., & Knauer, D. (2007). Brief mother-father-infant psychodynamic psychotherapy: Clinical and technical aspects. In M. Pozzi & B. Tydeman (eds.), *Innovations in Parent Infant Psychotherapy* 62–80. London: Karnac.

Panter-Brick, C., Burgess, A., Eggerman, M., McAllister, F., Pruett, K., & Leckman, J. (2014). Practitioner review: Engaging fathers – Recommendations for a game change in parenting interventions based on a systematic review of the global evidence. *Journal of Child Psychology and Psychiatry, and Allied Disciplines*, 55(11), 1187–212.

Papousek, M. (1987). Die Rolle des Vaters in der frühen Kindheit. *Ergebnisse der entwicklungspsychobiologischen Forschung. Kind und Umwelt*, 54, 29–49.

Paulson, J. F., & Bazemore, S. D. (2010). Prenatal and postpartum depression in fathers and its association with maternal depression. *Journal of the American Medical Association*, 303, 1961–69.

Perez, A. (2018). From pathological merger to a reflective, triangular space: Parent-infant psychotherapy with a mother with Borderline Personality Disorder. *Journal of Infant, Child and Adolescent Psychotherapy*, 17(1), 15–27.

Petfield, L., Startup, H., Droscher, H., & Cartwright-Hatton, S. (2015). Parenting in mothers with Borderline Personality Disorder and impact on child outcomes. *Evidence Based Mental Health*, 18(3), 67–75.

Petot, J.-M. (1990). *Melanie Klein: Vol. 1: First Discovery and First System (1919–1932)* (trans. C. Trollope). Madison, CT: International Universities Press.

Pruett, K. D., & Litzenberger, B. A. (1992). Latency development in children of primary nurturing fathers. Eight-year follow-up. *The Psychoanalytic Study of the Child*, 47, 85–101.

Paquette, D. (2004). Theorizing the father-child relationship: Mechanisms and developmental outcomes. *Human Development*, 47(4), 193–219.

Quinodoz, D. (1992). The psychoanalytic setting as the instrument of the container function. *International Journal of Psychoanalysis*, 73(4), 627–36.

Racker, H. (1982). *Transference and Countertransference*. London: Karnac.

Ramchandani, P., Stein, A., Evans, J., & O'Connor, T. G. (2005). Paternal depression in the postnatal period and child development: A prospective population study. *Lancet*, 365(9478), 2201–05. DOI: 10.1016/S0140-6736(05)66778-5.

Ramchandani, P. G., O'Connor, T. G., Evans, J., Heron, J., Murray, L., & Stein, A. (2008). The effects of pre- and postnatal depression in fathers: A natural experiment comparing the effects of exposure to depression on offspring. *Journal of Child Psychology and Psychiatry, and Allied Disciplines*, 49(10), 1069–78.

Ramchandani, P. G., Psychogiou, L., Vlachos, H., Iles, J., Sethna, V., Netsi, E., et al. (2011). Paternal depression: An examination of its links with father, child and family functioning in the postnatal period. *Depression and Anxiety*, 28(6), 471–77.

Raphael-Leff, J. (1985). Facilitators and regulators, participators and renouncers: Mothers and fathers orientations towards pregnancy and parenthood. *Journal of Psychosomatic Obstetrics & Gynaecology*, 4, 169–84.

Raphael-Leff, J. (1991). *Psychological Processes of Childbearing*. 4th Edition. London: Chapman & Hall, Anna Freud Centre, 2005.

Raphael-Leff, J. (1993). *Pregnancy – The Inside Story*. London: Sheldon Press; New York: Jason Aronson, 1996; London: Karnac, 2001.

Raphael-Leff, J. (2013). 'The intersubjective matrix': Influences on the independents' growth from 'object relations' to 'subject relations'. In S. Dermen, J. Keen, & P. Williams (eds.), *Contemporary Independent Psychoanalysis* (Chapter 3). London: Karnac Books.

Raphael-Leff, J. (2015). *The Dark Side of the Womb – Pregnancy, Parenting & Persecutory Anxieties*. London: Anna Freud Centre.

Rilling, K. K. (2013). The neural and hormonal bases of human parental care. *Neuropsychologia*, 51, 731–47.

Roopnarine, J. L., Fouts, H. N., Lamb, M. E., & Lewis-Elligan, T. Y. (2005). Mothers' and fathers' behaviors toward their 3 to 4-month-old infants in lower, middle, and upper socioeconomic African American families. *Developmental Psychology*, 41(5), 723–32.

Rosenfeld, H. (1987). Afterthought: Changing theories and changing techniques in psychoanalysis. In his *Impasse and Interpretation* 265–79. London: Tavistock Publications.

Ross, J. M. (1979). Fathering: A review of some psychoanalytic contributions on paternity. *The International Journal of Psycho-Analysis*, 60(Pt 3), 317–27.

Salomonsson, B. (1998). Between listening and expression: On desire, resonance and containment. *Scandinavian Psychoanalytic Review*, 21, 168–82.

Salomonsson, B. (2012). Has infantile sexuality anything to do with infants? *International Journal of Psychoanalysis*, 93(3), 631–47.

Salomonsson, B. (2013). Transferences in parent-infant psychoanalytic treatments. *International Journal of Psychoanalysis*, 94(4), 767–792.

Salomonsson, B. (2018a). *Psychodynamic Interventions in Pregnancy and Infancy: Clinical and Theoretical Perspectives*. London: Routledge.

Salomonsson, B. (2018b). Was Freud a Bionian? Perspectives from parent-infant psychoanalytic treatments. In A. Alisobhani & G. Corstorphine (eds.), *Everything We Know Nothing About: Explorations in Bion's 'O'*. London: Karnac.

Samuels, A. (1996). The good-enough father of whatever sex. In C. Clulow (ed.), *Partners Becoming Parents*. London: Sheldon Press.

Sander, L. W. (2002). Thinking differently: Principles of process in living systems and the specificity of being known. *Psychoanalytic Dialogues*, 12(1), 11–42.

Sandler, J. (1976). Countertransference and role-responsiveness. *International Review of Psychoanalysis*, 3, 43–47.

Sandler, J., & Sandler, A.-M. (1994). Phantasy and its transformations: A contemporary Freudian view. *International Journal of Psychoanalysis*, 75, 387–394.

Scheirs, J. G. M., & Bok, S. (2007). Psychological distress in caretakers or relatives of patients with Borderline Personality Disorder. *International Journal of Social Psychiatry*, 53(3), 195–203.

Schoppe-Sullivan, S. J., Altenburger, L. E., Settle, T. A., Kamp Dush, C. M., Sullivan, J. M., & Bower, D. J. (2014). Expectant fathers' intuitive parenting: Associations with parent characteristics and postpartum positive engagement. *Infant Mental Health Journal*, 35(5), 409–21.

Segal, H. (1989). Introduction. In J. Steiner (ed.), *The Oedipus Complex Today: Clinical Implications* 1–10. London: Karnac.

Spieler, S. (1984). Preoedipal girls need fathers. *Psychoanalytic Review*, 71(1), 63–80.

Spillius, E. B. (1983). Some developments from the work of Melanie Klein. *International Journal of Psychoanalysis*, 64, 321–332.

Stavrén-Eriksson, E. (2016). Transition to fatherhood in Sweden today (paper presented at a research student's course). Stockholm: Karolinska Institutet.

Steele, M., & Baradon, T. (2004). Clinical use of the adult attachment interview in parent-infant psychotherapy. *Infant Mental Health Journal*, 25(4), 284–99.

Stein, R. (1998). The enigmatic dimension of sexual experience: The 'otherness' of sexuality and primal seduction. *Psychoanalytic Quarterly*, 67, 594–625.

Stern, D. (2008). The clinical relevance of infancy: A progress report. *Infant Mental Health Journal*, 29(3), 177–88. DOI: 10.1002/imhj.

Stern, D. N. (1995). *The Motherhood Constellation*. New York: Basic Books.

Stoller, R. J. (1994). *Sex and Gender: The Development of Masculinity and Femininity.* London: Karnac Books.

Straker, G. (2006). The anti-analytic third. *The Psychoanalytic Review*, 93(5), 729–53.

Swain, J. E., Dayton, C. J., Kim, P., Tolman, R. M., & Volling, B. L. (2014). Progress on the paternal brain: Theory, animal models, human brain research, and mental health implications. *Infant Mental Health Journal*, 35, 394–408. DOI: 10.1002/imhj.21471.

Target, M., & Fonagy, P. (2000). Playing with reality: III. The persistence of dual psychic reality in borderline patients. *The International Journal of Psychoanalysis*, 81(5), 853–73.

Target, M., & Fonagy, P. (2002). Fathers in modern psychoanalysis and in society: The role of the father and child development. In J. Trowell & A. Etchegoyen (eds.), *The Importance of Fathers – A Psychoanalytic Re-evaluation* 45–66. Hove: Brunner-Routledge.

Thomson-Salo, F., & Paul, C. (2007). *The Baby as Subject*. 2nd Edition. Melbourne: The University of Melbourne and Royal Children's Hospital.

van IJzendoorn, M. (1995). Adult attachment representations, parental responsiveness, and infant attachment: A meta-analysis on the predictive validity of the adult attachment interview. *Psychological Bulletin*, 117(3), 387–403.

von Bertalanffy, K. L. (1968). *General System Theory: Foundations, Development, Applications*. New York: George Braziller.

Widlöcher, D. (2002). *Infantile Sexuality and Attachment*. New York: Other Press.

Winnicott, D. W. (1949). Hate in the counter-transference. *International Journal of Psychoanalysis*, 30, 69–74.

Winnicott, D. W. (1949/1988). *Babies and Their Mothers*. London: Free Association Books.

Winnicott, D. W. (1956). Primary maternal preoccupation. In D. W. Winnicott (ed.), *Through Pediatrics to Psychoanalysis* 300–05. London: Tavistock Publications, New York: Basic books, 1958.

Winnicott, D. W. (1960). The theory of the parent-infant relationship. In D. W. Winnicott (ed.), *The Maturational Processes in the Theory of Emotional Development* 37–55. Madison, WI: International Universities Press.

Winnicott, D. W. (1961). Varieties of psychotherapy. In *The Collected Works of Donald Winnicott*, Vol. 6, 197–204. New York: Oxford University Press, (2016).

Winnicott, D. W. (1964). What about fathers. In his *The Child, the Family and the Outside World* 113–18.

Winnicott, D. W. (1965). A child psychiatry case illustrating delayed reaction to loss. In *The Collected Works of Donald Winnicott*, Vol. 6, 279–304. New York: Oxford University Press, 2016.

Wong, Y. J., Ho, M.-H. R., Wang, S.-Y., & Miller, I. S. K. (2017). Meta-analyses of the relationship between conformity to masculine norms and mental health-related outcomes. *Journal of Counseling Psychology*, 64, 80–93.

Woodhead, J. (2004). Shifting triangles: Images of father in sequences from parent-infant psychotherapy. *Infant Observation*, 7(2&3), 76–90.

Yogman, M. Y. (1982). Observations on the father-infant relationship. In S. Cath, A. Gurwitt, & J. M. Ross (eds.), *Father and Child: Developmental and Clinical Perspectives* 101–22. Boston, MA: Little & Brown & Co.

Zamanian, K. (2011). Attachment theory as defense: What happened to infantile sexuality? *Psychoanalytic Psychology*, 28(1), 33–47.

Zeuthen, K., & Gammelgaard, J. (2010). Infantile sexuality – The concept, its history and place in contemporary psychoanalysis. *Scandinavian Psychoanalytic Review*, 33(1), 3–12.

Index

abandonment 99, 119, 121, 122–3
Abelin, E. L. 15
Abell, S. C. 24
absent fathers 22–3, 39, 44–5, 48, 52, 99, 104
abuse 45, 98, 118, 119
abusive/violent fathers 50–3, 54, 57–63, 70, 104, 152, 167–8, 171
adolescence 16, 167
Adult Attachment Interview (AAI) 30–1, 43
affect regulation 25; *see also* emotion regulation
African Americans 16–17
agency 11, 69, 101; generative 64, 67, 79
aggression 101, 125–6, 127, 130, 167; *see also* abusive/violent fathers
Allison, E. 42
ambivalence 71, 74, 76, 167–8, 169–70
anger 57, 143; abusive partners 61; borderline personality disorder couple 40, 45, 46, 48; male therapists 100, 103, 104; relationship breakdowns 99; self-harm 61; therapist's 115, 156
Anna Freud National Centre for Children and Families 1, 39, 86
anxiety 53, 64, 69–70, 102, 109–10; borderline personality disorder couple 40; defensive sexual transference 115, 116; Freud 127; paternal orientations 71–2, 74; separation 72, 157; sexuality 91
anxiety disorder 53
après coup 29, 38
attachment 9, 10, 16, 20, 82n7; borderline personality disorder couples 41; forbidden 40; positive affect arousal 18; unresolved loss 34
attraction 51, 52, 59, 102, 143, 152
Atzil, S. 17
autism 131–2, 136–7
avoidance 109

Baradon, Tessa 85–93, 143, 147–8, 154, 156–7, 161–4, 166, 169–71
Barrows, P. 119
bed wetting 37
beliefs 64, 65
Belsky, J. 89
bereavement 8, 28–9, 30–8, 45, 150, 159, 161–2
Bergbom, I. 145
Bevington, Dickon 1–13, 169
Bion, W. R. 24, 117, 123
birth 5–7, 29, 72–3
birth rates 79–80
bisexuality 26, 77
bodies 25
Bollas, C. 164
borderline personality disorder 39–49, 158–9, 167
Bouchard, S. 41
boundaries 73, 143
Bowlby, John 78, 82n7
boys 24, 26, 101, 131, 134, 138, 167–8
brain regions 17
breast 14, 24, 164, 166
breastfeeding 70, 72, 75, 76, 91–2, 109
Britton, Ronald 14, 42, 120, 123, 139

Cairo, S. 21
Campbell, C. 42
Carneiro, C. 21
castration 14, 130
child-bearing 68
child development 14–27, 39

child protection 60
childcare 65, 75–6, 78, 80n1, 81n4, 83n8, 83n9
co-parenting 65, 77, 81n5; interventions 161; male therapists 94, 97, 98, 99, 104
communication: communication failures 42; nonverbal 112–13; triadic relationships 89
compassion 74
'completely at-a-loss-ness' 1–2
'conflicted' orientation 64, 71, 75
conflicts: borderline personality disorder couples 41; male therapists 97; Oedipal 120; parental 22, 89; triangular 168
'contagious resonance' 65, 69, 71
container/contained 117, 123
containment 77, 139, 148, 149
cooperative baby-care 65
coping mechanisms 71, 72, 73
Corboz-Warnery, A. 21
countertransference 23, 93, 150–1, 156–7, 163; awareness of 160; borderline personality disorder couple 158; cultural bias 109, 111–12; emotional attunement 54; Freud 140; male therapists 102, 143; negative 106, 113–16
couple relationship 90, 117–23; couple intimacy 81n5; interventions 161, 163; male therapists 97, 98
Cowan, P. A. and C. P. 89
cultural bias 95, 106–12
cultural conventions 83n11

Daley, M. 22
damaging father 39, 45
Davids, M. F. 20
Davies, N. 24–5, 43
Dayton, C. J. 17
death 28–9; *see also* bereavement
defences 50–1, 106, 146, 151, 169; childhood bereavement 28–9, 31–2, 35–6, 37, 38, 159, 162; mothers 52–3, 55–6, 58–9, 62, 63; new parents 69; 'Renouncers' 72; unconscious 163; violent fathers 60–1
demographic changes 78–80
denial 50, 51, 59, 60–1, 62
depression 53, 60, 82n5, 89–90; paternal 19, 111; postnatal 18–19, 39, 87, 98
depressive position 14, 20
Diamond, Michael J. 139
Dickstein, S. 22
differentiation 15
discipline 118, 119, 128
disorganised attachment 34, 42
dissociation 72
drive theory 20
dual-income families 75
Dugmore, N. 96
Durkheim, E. 79
dyadic relationships 24, 85, 88, 90–1, 94, 170; *see also* mother-infant relationship

Eagle, G. 24–5, 43
early child development 14–27
ego 15, 140
ego psychology 152
Eizirik, C. L. 139
Emanuel, Louise 90, 117–23, 149, 163
emotion regulation 46, 48; *see also* affect regulation
emotional climate 65, 75
emotional dysregulation 41, 42, 43
emotions 65, 143; 'Reciprocators' 74; therapist's 112, 113–16
empathy 6, 74, 93, 136
enactments 41, 96, 97
engulfment 15, 64, 77, 127, 130, 170
enmeshment 39, 41–2, 45–6, 47, 48, 100, 158; *see also* merger
environmental provision 85
eroticised feelings 100, 103, 104–5, 112, 113, 116
Etchegoyen, A. 15–16
exclusion: borderline personality disorder couple 167; children 119–20, 121–2, 163; fathers 93, 95, 97, 98–9, 112, 167; male therapists 96; mothers 164–5; triadic relationships 89; triangular 143
expectation of fatherhood 2–4

'Facilitator' mothers 75–6
Fagin, Abel 94–105, 142–3, 170
failure 1, 66, 98, 170; failing gracefully 1, 8, 12, 169; fear of 9
Faimberg, H. 150
family alliance 21–2
family relationships 4–5
family therapy 162
fantasies: aggressive 101; childhood bereavement 29, 34, 36, 38; damaging father 39, 45; Freud 141; male therapists

96; 'motherhood constellation' 107; omniscience 132; paternal orientations 71; persecutory 89; sexualised 92–3; transition to fatherhood 69; unconscious 149, 155; *see also* phantasies
Fast, Irene 66
'father hunger' 27, 101, 163
fatherhood: anxiety 69–70; cultural bias 106; demographic changes 78–80; expectation of 2–4; as expression of emotion 65; 'fatherhood constellation' 108, 109, 116, 146; Freud on 67–8; generations 65–6; neurobiology of 17; paternal orientations 64–5, 70–7, 79, 80; single fatherhood by choice 78; transition to 68–9, 108, 144
fathers: absent 22–3, 39, 44–5, 48, 52, 99, 104; agreed frame for engagement 86; assertive 145–6; borderline personality disorder couple 39–49, 158–9, 167; childhood bereavement 28–9, 30–8, 150, 159, 161–2; concept of 'father' 68; cultural bias 106–12; defensive processes 50–1; difficulties fulfilling the paternal function 125–38; father-focused interventions 161–2; 'father transference' 156–7, 160; Freud's view 139–41, 144, 149; internal father 16, 23–7, 45, 82n7; male therapists 94, 95, 104; mother's influence on 169; partner dynamics 81n5; paternal engagement 67–8; paternal orientations 64–5, 70–7, 79, 80; perinatal disturbance 82n5; play 77; real 15–16, 82n7, 124–5, 129, 130, 170; relationship breakdowns 98–9; role in early child development 14–27; sexual tensions 112–16; triadic relationships 19–23, 85–93, 147–8, 164–8; violent/abusive 50–3, 54, 57–63, 70, 98, 104, 152, 167–8, 171; working 'in the presence of' 87–8; working with father-baby dyads 88; *see also* paternal function
Favez, N. 21–2
fear 8; abusive partners 61; borderline personality disorder couple 45, 46; of failure 9; mothers 58; 'Renouncers' 73
Feldman, R. 17, 18
femininity 108, 135, 168, 171
feminism 64, 82n7
Ferenczi, S. 150
Field, T. 18
Fivaz, Elisabeth 20–2
Fonagy, P. 20, 25, 41, 42
Ford, Gina 33, 159
forgiveness 13
Fouts, H. N. 16
Freud, Anna 28, 152, 165
Freud, Hendrika 152
Freud, Sigmund 14, 124, 139–41, 148, 149; bisexuality 26, 77; childhood 66; fatherhood 67–8; Little Hans 125, 126; mourning 28; paternal substitutes 127; repetition compulsion 53; sexual difference 145; sexuality 144; transference 155
frustration tolerance 25
Furman, Erna 28–9, 38

gaze transitions 21, 22
gender 25, 26; gender 66, 81n2; gender equality discourse 131; gender roles 24, 80, 83n11; male therapists 94, 95–6, 104–5; normative gender expectations 67
generations 65–6
generative agency 64, 67, 79
generative identity 66, 67, 69, 71
Genesoni, L. 144–5
girls 24, 26
Golombok, S. 77
Goodman, S. H. 19
Gosliner, B. 15
grandiosity 12
Green, A. 23–4, 25
Greenacre, P. 67
guilt 102, 104; borderline personality disorder couple 39, 43–4, 46, 48–9, 158–9; childhood bereavement 29, 35, 38; damaging father 45; 'Participators' 72; self-harm 61

Helmuth, Hug 165
helplessness 53, 98, 104, 170; boundaries 143; childhood bereavement 32, 33; failure of paternal function 128, 129; Freud 140, 141; parents 123
Hendler, T. 17
Herzog, J. M. 17, 26–7, 101
homosexuality 77, 79; *see also* same-sex couples
hopelessness 40, 53, 60
Hopkins, J. 54
hormones 82n6

identification 14, 91, 93, 108, 166; with baby 107; generative identity 67; 'Participators' 71–2, 74; transgender 81n2; *see also* projective identification
identity: borderline personality disorder couple 48; child's 15; family relationships 5; gender 66, 81n2; generative 66, 67, 69, 71; male 78, 108–9, 116, 146; parenting 76
'iGeneration' 66
impotence 69
individuation 15, 23
infant-focused interventions 161, 162–3
'infantile prototypes' 155
infantile sexuality 143–4, 146, 148
insecure attachment 41
instinct theory 20
intergenerational transmission 53, 57, 71, 111–12, 150, 152
internal father 16, 23–7, 45, 82n7
intersubjectivity 26–7
interventions 161–4
intimacy 9, 64, 170; couple 81n5; male therapists 96, 100, 102; marital relationship 119; therapeutic encounter 91

Jaques, Elliott 78
jealousy 70, 73, 111, 120, 143, 146
Jones, Amanda 50–63, 150, 151–2, 163, 167–8, 170–1
Joseph, B. 155
Joyce, Angela 28–38, 150–1, 159, 161–2, 170

Kernberg, O. 23
Kestenberg, Judith 66
Kim, P. 17
Klein, Melanie 14, 66, 149, 155, 165
Klitzing, Kai von 14–27, 90, 139, 141, 146, 148, 154, 164–8, 169
Knauer, D. 89
Kramer, S. 82n7

Lacan, J. 124, 130, 144, 148; aggressiveness 127; father as third person 14–15, 67–8; Little Hans 125, 129
Lamb, M. E. 16
language 11, 15
Laplanche, J. 165
Larkin, Philip 1
latency 35
Lausanne Trilogue Play 20–1, 22
Layland, Ralph 74–5
Laznik, Marie-Christie 124–38, 141–2, 163, 168, 170
Lebovici, S. 17, 20, 165
lesbians 68–9, 136, 141; *see also* same-sex couples
Lewis-Elligan, T. Y. 16
libidinal group 90–1
libido 100
Liebman, S. J. 24
Lindwall, L. 145
long-term psychotherapeutic work 153
loss: childhood bereavement 28–9, 30–1, 37, 38, 45; male therapists 100; Oedipal rivalry 120; unresolved 34
love 9, 10, 19, 140, 146
Lundgren, I. 145
Lusby, C. M. 19
Luyten, P. 42

Mahler, Margret 15, 66
male therapists 94–105, 142–3
Mann, D. 102
masculinity 78–9, 80, 145, 146
maternal function 117–18, 148, 149, 163
maternal orientations 75–6
McDougall, Joyce 29, 38
McHale, J. 22, 94
Mead, M. 106
media 78, 79
Melman, Charles 138
memories 13, 61
MenCare Global Fatherhood campaign 83n9
mental representations 22
mentalisation 23, 42, 48, 62, 97, 164, 170
merger 39, 41–2, 43, 47, 119, 170; *see also* enmeshment
milestones 11
Millennials 66
mistrust 42, 45, 104, 158
Modh, C. 145
mother-infant relationship 146, 148; cultural bias 106–7, 109; dyadic mother-infant psychotherapy 90–1; exclusion of father 95; intimacy with newborn 9; male therapists 96, 99–102; positive affect 18
'motherhood constellation' 90–1, 107, 146, 171
mothers 169–71; availability of 16–17; borderline personality disorder couple

39, 40, 41–3, 45–8, 158–9, 167; childhood bereavement 30, 32–6, 37, 38; critical 57; dyadic mother-infant psychotherapy 90–1; Green on 24; identification with 108; law of the mother 131; male therapists 95, 99–104; maternal function 117–18, 148, 149, 163; maternal orientations 75–6; maternal transference 156, 157; mother-focused interventions 161, 162; omniscience 132, 135; partner dynamics 81n5; paternal function performed by 141; 'phallic' 135, 168, 170; play 77; psychoanalytic theory 14, 20, 64, 77, 82n7; relationship breakdowns 98–9; serious mental illness 50, 51, 53, 61; therapeutic work without the father 51–63, 152; triadic relationships 20, 22–3, 85–93, 147–8, 164–8; Winnicott on 15, 18, 107
mourning 28–9, 35, 38, 146, 157, 159

narcissism 5, 72, 89, 124, 140
neglect 45
neurobiology 17
neurosis 14
Newport, D. J. 19
nom du père 15, 132, 138, 168, 170
non du père 15, 168
nonverbal communication 112–13
Novick, K. K. and J. 165

object constancy 28, 38
object relations 20, 77, 109, 164
obsessive compulsive disorder 53
Oedipal anxieties 96, 97
Oedipal period 19, 23–4
Oedipal resolution 120, 130
Oedipus complex 14, 35–6, 70, 124, 126, 129, 140
omnipotence 67, 80, 123, 134, 149, 170
omnipotent control 50, 51, 58–9, 60–1, 62
omniscience 132, 135

pain 5–6
Palacio Espasa, F. 89
Papousek, M. 18
Paquette, D. 17
parent-child triad *see* triadic relationships
parental leave 70, 81n1, 81n4
parenting 1–2, 7, 163; changes in parenting paradigms 64; couple relationship 117, 118; generative identity 66; intuitive behaviours 18; multifactorial nature of 65; predetermined responses 145
parents, internal 52–3
'Participator' fathers 64, 71–2, 74, 75, 76
paternal function 64, 77, 124–38, 141, 149, 168; borderline personality disorder couple 46, 48; boundaries 143; containment of mother-infant dyad 148; couple relationships 117–18; four dimensions 25, 43; internalisation of parental object 163; male therapists 103; therapist's role 90; triangulation 82n7
paternal orientations 64–5, 70–7, 79, 80
Patriarchy 67
penis 24
penis envy 14
Perez, Alejandra 39–49, 152–3, 158–9, 162–3, 167, 170
personality disorders 41
'phallic' mothers 135, 168, 170
phallic rivalry 37
phantasies 26, 95, 100, 165, 170; *see also* fantasies
Phares, V. 94
physiological responses 76, 82n6
play 16, 17, 26, 77, 166; borderline personality disorder couple 45; *Lausanne Trilogue Play* 20–1, 22; positive affect arousal 18; rough-and-tumble 24; triad-focused interventions 164
positive affect 18
postnatal depression 18–19, 39, 87, 98
Prall, R. 82n7
pregnancy 2–4, 16, 69; paternal anxiety 70; paternal orientations 71, 72, 74
primary maternal preoccupation 107
projection 50, 54, 167–8, 171; abusive/violent fathers 59, 60–1, 62; mentalisation thwarted by 62; mothers 57, 58, 62; working with the triad 89, 93
projective identification 20, 41, 72, 164
'psychoanalytic mindfulness' 96
psychoanalytic theory 23, 64, 77, 82n7; *après coup* 29; mother-infant relationship 106–7; mourning 28, 35; parent-child triad 19–20; repetition compulsion 53; restricted role of father 139; theories of early development 14; transference 155; triadic relationships 24–5; unconscious processes 53; *see also* Freud
psychosexual distinction 66

Raphael-Leff, Joan 64–84, 144–5, 169
'Reciprocator' fathers 64, 73–4, 76
'Reciprocator' mothers 75–6
reciprocity 9
reflective capacity 36
'Regulator' mothers 75–6
relationship breakdowns 98–9, 101
'Renouncer' fathers 64, 72–3, 74, 75–7
reparative male figure, therapist as 98–100
repetition compulsion 53, 171
repression 38
responsibility, 'time-span' of parental 64
reverie 91
risk assessment 51
rituals 7–8
Robertson, J. 22
Roopnarine, J. L. 16
rules 33, 159

safeguarding 60
Salomonsson, Björn 90, 139–53, 154–61, 162
same-sex couples 68–9, 75, 77, 83n10; *see also* lesbians
Sandler, J. and A.-M. 155
Scaiola, C. L. 21
Schoppe-Sullivan, S. J. 18
Segal, Hanna 120
Segal, Yael 106–16, 139, 145–6, 156, 170
self 23, 26, 39, 71, 73–4; *see also* identity
self-discovery 66, 76
self-harm 61
separation 14, 15, 43, 48, 119, 169
separation anxiety 72, 157
serious mental illness 50, 51, 53, 61
sexism 79
sexual belligerence 70
sexual desire 100, 102, 156
sexual difference 66–7, 68, 145
sexual intercourse 50, 52, 93
sexualisation 92–3, 102, 109, 112–16, 156
sexuality 26, 141, 145–6, 166–7; drive/instinct theory 20; infantile 143–4, 146, 148; male therapists 142–3; parental 120; working with the triad 91–3, 148
siblings 55, 58, 61, 91, 120
single fatherhood 78, 83n8
socioeconomic status 16–17
sperm decline 80
splitting 32, 50, 168, 170; abusive/violent fathers 60–1; infants 20; mentalisation thwarted by 62; 'Renouncers' 72; triadic relationships 89
Spock, Benjamin 78
Stavrén-Eriksson, E. 142
Stern, Daniel 85, 107, 108, 151
Stowe, Z. N. 19
stress 89
superego 130
supervision 115, 116
Swain, J. E. 17
symbolisation 23
symbols 15

Tallandini, M. A. 144–5
tantrums 118
Target, M. 20, 25, 41
Tavistock Clinic 81n2, 117
therapeutic alliance 46, 102, 161
therapeutic encounter 86, 91, 96, 100, 102, 170
the third 25, 164, 166, 170; analyst as 23; father as third person 14–15, 20; paternal function 90, 130, 136; 'third position' 123; 'thirdness' 24, 82n7
Thompson, K. 19
'time-span' of parental responsibility 64
Tolman, R. M. 17
transference 23, 112, 140, 154–61; childhood bereavement 32, 38; definition of 154–5; dyadic mother-infant psychotherapy 90–1; male therapists 96, 97, 100–1, 102, 103, 104, 143; maternal 156; negative 149, 156, 157, 160; transference-love 113–16; *see also* countertransference
trauma 29, 57, 95, 96–7, 119, 150
triadic relationships 19–23, 24, 27, 164–8; male therapists 94, 96–8; triad-focused interventions 161, 163–4; triadic attachment 82n7; triadic capacity of therapist 165, 166; working with the triad 85–93, 96–8, 147–8
triangulation 15–16, 119–20, 154, 164; borderline personality disorder couple 46, 167; Fivaz group 20–2; good enough father 165; inhibition of 169; interventions 161, 162; Kernberg 23; paternal function 25, 82n7
Truby King, Frederic 78

umbilical cord 7–8
uncertainty 1, 74

the unconscious 24, 155
unconscious processes 53
urbanisation 79

values 71, 94, 106, 112
violent/abusive fathers 50–3, 54, 57–63, 70, 98, 104, 152, 167–8, 171
Volling, B. L. 17, 89

walking 11
Winetraub, Y. 17
Winnicott, D. W. 15, 24, 41, 108, 169; childcare 78; childhood bereavement 29; gatekeeping role of mother 18; maternal environmental provision 85; primary maternal preoccupation 107
withdrawal 90, 163, 165; borderline personality disorder couple 40, 41, 43–4, 46–8; mothers 59; 'Renouncers' 72
women: borderline personality disorder 41; demographic changes 79–80; professionals 94; *see also* mothers

Yeats, W. B. 10

Zagoory-Sharon, O. 17

For Product Safety Concerns and Information please contact our EU representative GPSR@taylorandfrancis.com
Taylor & Francis Verlag GmbH, Kaufingerstraße 24, 80331 München, Germany

www.ingramcontent.com/pod-product-compliance
Ingram Content Group UK Ltd.
Pitfield, Milton Keynes, MK11 3LW, UK
UKHW020202200926
475702UK00004B/578
9781138093423